THINENOUGH

THIN**ENOUGH**

My Spiritual Journey
Through the Living Death
of an Eating Disorder

By Sheryle Cruse

n e w
hope
PUBLISHERS

Birmingham, Alabama

New Hope® Publishers
P. O. Box 12065
Birmingham, AL 35202-2065
www.newhopepublishers.com

Library of Congress Cataloging-in-Publication Data

Cruse, Sheryle, 1971-
  Thin enough : my spiritual journey through the living death of an eating disorder / by Sheryle Cruse.
    p. cm.
  Includes bibliographical references.
  ISBN 1-59669-003-8 (softcover)
  1. Cruse, Sheryle, 1971- 2. Eating disorders—Patients—Religious life. 3. Eating disorders— Religious aspects—Christianity. I. Title.
  BV4910.35.C78 2006
  248.8'61968526—dc22
          2005029230

This book is intended to be a resource and help on the subject of eating disorders and to point the reader to the source materials that contain a more thorough treatment of the subject. None of the information presented in this book is meant to be a prescription for any kind of treatment, medical or otherwise, and reference to other organizations and materials is for convenience only and is not intended as an endorsement. The author has made every effort to present the current research accurately and assumes no responsibility for inaccuracies, omissions, or errors contained in the source materials. The author and publisher are not liable for misuse of the information provided. The author and publisher are neither liable nor responsible to any person or entity for any loss, damage, injury, or death caused or alleged to be caused by the information in this book.

ISBN: 1-59669-003-8

N064130 • 0206 • 9M1

Dedication

This is dedicated

to every girl

who struggles with herself,

her eating, her body, and her God.

There *is* hope

that things will get better.

"Little girl, I say to you, arise."
—Mark 5:41

Table of Contents

Acknow**ledge**ments

Many thanks to those who made this book—this dream—possible.

First, I'd like to thank my three agents of divine intervention, love, and involvement. Without you three especially, this book would be frustrated pages shoved in a bottom drawer, covered in dust.

To my mother, Genevieve: Thank you for being the first "woman of God" in my life, for your constant and patient prayers and love.

To my husband, my constant friend, and my computer wiz, Russell: Thank you for being my steady "S" man, for helping me through every tedious and difficult step, both with the eating disorders and with the book itself.

To my spiritual mentor, "editor," and guide, Pastor Tom Taylor: Thank you for your prayers, support, and belief that this could ever be a book in the first place—and then helping me get through it all.

Additional thanks

To my friends and family for their love, prayers, and support, for Pastors Larry and Tiz Huch and the entire New Beginnings Christian Center family in Portland, Oregon, and Dallas/Fort Worth, Texas.

To every person and organization who graciously granted me permission to include their valuable and helpful resources for eating disorder sufferers.

To my editor, Rebecca England, and all of the incredible staff at New Hope Publishers.

Introduction

It was twelve o' clock midnight, and the alarm blared.

"Get up! You must do this!" yelled a voice from somewhere deep within me. Slowly rising from my bed, I avoided the light-headed dizziness and concentrated on every movement.

Already exhausted, I began this day as I did most others, with a collapsing spell. Thud! "How many calories are burned in a drop thud anyway?" I thought to myself as I accepted the collapse as a part of my routine. It was merely the price I had to pay to be 19 years old, 5 feet 4 inches tall, and 80 pounds. That kind of thinness wouldn't happen unless I *made* it happen!

I obeyed my inner drill sergeant and stumbled in the dark to my exercise equipment. In the beginning, I had enjoyed the sense of accomplishment, the toned body, and the natural endorphin-high that exercise brought me. Somehow that had morphed into the morning installment of my daily punishment.

Driven by fear, I believed my critical inner voice when it told me things such as:

> *No one will ever want you unless you're thin, beautiful, and perfect, you know!*
>
> *You're not good enough! Who do you think you're kidding by doing this? But you'd better not stop!*
>
> *You have to finish this. You won't be able to live with yourself if you don't.*

The next six punishing hours became a thud fest. I tried to find the emotional strength to deal with my inner commandant's orders and enough physical strength to keep from fainting again. Collapsing was inevitable, though. I saw it as the price I needed to pay to have perfection and worth.

Each morning, I dreaded and feared the fainting. I knew it would happen. Would I be out for three seconds, thirty seconds, or thirty minutes this morning? I tried to control where I fainted. When I couldn't, I'd collapse on the equipment, hitting my head on a barbell or bike pedal. Would my mother discover me lying on the floor? I didn't want to face her "I'm surprised you're still alive" comments. I prayed not to get caught.

I was fortunate this morning. I was only out for a few seconds. "Okay, now," I coached myself, "come up slowly from the floor." I tried to make no sudden movements as I crawled from the family room into the kitchen. I was a picture of dignity and self-empowerment.

I didn't like it, but I knew I had to eat something, just enough to keep myself from "thudding" repeatedly.

Dazed and weak, I devoted my brainpower to counting the calories of foods that were safe. Foods in the 15 to 50 calories-per-serving range, like ketchup, jams, and jelly, were okay. Besides, they had sugar, so I saw them as "treats." I may have been near death, antifood, and sick, but I still had my sweet tooth. I crawled to the fridge, opened the door, and chose a jar of strawberry jam. "There!" I thought, as I jammed my bony fingers into the bottom crevices of the jar, digging out finger-scoops of this safe food. "That'll show Mom I am eating something!"

As I sat on the kitchen floor, the open refrigerator door provided the only light in the room. I didn't want to draw attention to what I was doing. I hovered over that jar of strawberry jam, obsessing about how much I could eat before my stomach felt too full and too fat. I also was racing against time, trying to finish before my family woke up. But for a moment, all that mattered was strawberry jam.

"Whoa! Way too much! You just need enough to get through the day. Keep going and you're going to get fat!" I told myself this repeatedly. And so I stopped and squelched my self-indulgence, while relocating my self-control. I put away the jam and shut the fridge door. Now what?

Damage assessment: Where would the jam show up on me? I panicked. I had to know. I had chosen to eat it, now I chose to face the consequences.

I stumbled back to my bedroom and timidly faced the truth. "There's no use crying over spilled milk." (Even my self-mocking had food references in it.) "You chose to eat this. You have no one to blame but yourself!"

I looked in the mirror and saw why I chose to put myself through all of this. There it was: my skeleton body, all 80 pounds of it. I was relieved to see that I was still okay; I hadn't eaten too much after all. I continued staring, admiring my golden rib cage, my trophy. It stuck out and seemed sharp enough to stab someone, almost breaking out of my skin.

I had sculpted myself into my own thin, perfect creation. I had proven everybody wrong. I wasn't just a fat, lumpy girl! I felt vindicated. Starvation, perfection, and destruction were the mandates I had given myself. Wasting away meant that I was pretty, worthy, and somehow *holy*. I couldn't stop.

I stood in my bedroom in front of my three-way mirror. I'd seen so many versions of myself. I'd been fat and thin, feeling both unworthy and worthy. Yet I was never satisfied.

I strained to continue staring in my mirror, dizzy. Demons of discontent, failure, and constant want reflected back at me. I felt myself falling to the floor as my vision turned black. Fainting was a welcome escape. Unconscious, I didn't have to think about how fat I was, how much I wanted food, how much God hated me, or how much I wanted it all to end. Each time

I woke up, I wanted to just lie there on the floor instead. Life was too difficult and too painful. I wanted to die. How much worse could this get?

I was left alone with questions I couldn't answer. "What should I do then when I'm hungry?" "What should I do when I can never get full?" Unable to answer any of these questions, I longed for the past. I missed my childhood innocence, when answers came so simply. You eat when you're hungry, and you believe that God loves you. I missed having those simple answers, and I thought I'd never have them again. I never dreamed that God would use all of this to show me that His love is real, even for this broken girl.

Chapter One

Stuffed Unconscious

Stuffed Unconscious (Feast Unaware)

The little girl reached out arms for love,
and with arms returning empty
She asked herself,
"What *can* I have?"
The little girl looked all around
and food answered her,
smirking smile
on plate after plate,
She gave it the voice
to tell her,
"I love you"
because
she didn't think anyone
did-would-could,
She heard the food
speak to her
first
in loving, soothing
comfort
every sensation
every touch
love was in every bite
she took,

so she took
more and more
hoping
she'd be filled up
enough,
Feast after feast
she thought
would release her
to the high comfort
of being full,
The little girl kept feeding
Too much,
never enough,
Stuffed unconscious
Feast unaware—
At the end of every spoon-fed feast—
emptiness
No matter how much she ate
She couldn't get full,
And she was left with only
a bitter taste
and a regret
that was
her
fat
unacceptable
body.

It's so simple being a child. When I was a little girl, Jesus was real to me, and I knew He loved me. One of my clearest, earliest memories was watching a television mini-series on Jesus. It sealed the deal for my falling in love with Him. The story of Jairus's daughter (**Mark 5:35–43**) really stuck out to me. I identified with the little girl that Jesus brought back to life, probably because she was a young girl just like me. When Jesus touched her, healed her, hugged her, and loved her, I wanted to be her. I wanted to love Jesus and be that close to Him. I had a simple, childlike faith. I was an innocent, *pre*apple Eve. I was *pre*hurt and *pre*scarred. But I grew up, and I ate the apple.

When did my childlike faith change? It's difficult to say. Like a lot of people, I come from a long line of family members who have turned to lies and assorted addictions to escape their painful lives. Secrecy, denial, lies, and desperate attempts at escape were my family's typical answers. I was born into a family where abusive behavior was called "discipline," and if you got love and affection you were "being spoiled." A long line of family members learned what they lived—abuse—and accepted it as their lot in life. Although they tried their best, generation after generation raised children without knowing how to love them. Parenting consisted of a yell, temper tantrum, or "silent treatment" here, and a smack, threat, or a "whupping" there.

This family model taught me the meaning of "father." Drawing conclusions from the perspective of a three-, four-, or five-year-old, I believed this must be how a father treated his child. My dad first defined what both fathers and men represented to me. Therefore, logically, I imagined God to be this kind of father, too. He must not love or want me either. I took it further from there and began to feel that God was angry with me and even hated me. I decided in my little-girl mind right then and there that I was a wrong, "bad little girl." Not hurt, not sad, not confused—just wrong.

> *"Since you were precious in My sight . . .*
> *I have loved you."*
> *—Isaiah 43:4*

Although I was taught that God loved me, I wasn't taught that God wanted to help me. I was completely in the dark about the fact that I could go to God—my Father—and He'd help me. As a little girl, I didn't know that He could erase the pain that I was going through, healing and completing me with His love. I only knew two things—that I was somehow "wrong" and definitely all alone. Do you see where this is going? I needed someone, something (God), but I found a substitute instead. Food.

Question: Does food make you feel happy and calm?

You know the saying, "Misery loves company"? Well, misery loves food, too. I was hurt, rejected, miserable, but unaware of it. I knew that I wanted love, but when I reached out, food was always there instead. When "quality time" with my parents wasn't there, food was never too busy. When hugs, kisses, affection, and compliments weren't there, food was close by. Candy, chocolate, cookies, and ice cream were there to sweeten my lonely tears. Pot pies, mashed potatoes, hamburgers, and fries were there to nurture and warm me whenever I felt a cold, distant rejection. Pretzels, potato chips, and anything salty or crunchy provided welcome relief from frustration. I could just crunch it away. I had a food for every reason and a reason for every food. Comfort food—that's what it was all about. Who needed a mother, father, other people, or God? They only disappoint and hurt you. I had food. And so, I ate.

At first it was cute, I suppose. The chubby little cheeks, the round stomach, and the baby fat—it was tolerated for a while, but eventually, the grace ran out. Because food was her chosen drug, her chosen addiction, Mom had battled her own "weight problem" her entire life. She was alarmed to see the dreaded sin manifesting itself in her little girl. It was time to fix the problem. It was time to fix me. When she saw her coping mechanism reflected in me, she introduced me to my first diet. I was seven years old.

I remember Mom coaxing me into my first diet. All I ate for days straight was pineapple. Al-o-o-ha! It took me at least a good 10 to 15 years before I could enjoy the fruit again. But I trusted Mom. She knew best. After all, I'd seen her go on many diets before. I thought, "If I do this, then I'll be okay. If I do this, then I'll make things better." A diet was the answer.

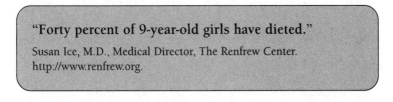

"Forty percent of 9-year-old girls have dieted."
Susan Ice, M.D., Medical Director, The Renfrew Center.
http://www.renfrew.org.

I didn't know then that God was already the answer. I didn't know that when God looked at me, He saw more than a chubby little girl with chubby cheeks, a chubby stomach, and chubby legs. I didn't know that He saw His little girl, His daughter, whom He *loved*.

Preventing Obesity: Tips for Parents

- Respect your child's appetite: Children do not need to finish every bottle or meal.

- Avoid preprepared and sugared foods when possible.

- Limit the amount of high-calorie foods kept in the home.

- Provide a healthy diet, with 30 percent or fewer calories derived from fat.

- Provide ample fiber in the child's diet.

- Skim milk may safely replace whole milk at two years of age.

- Do not provide food for comfort or as a reward.

- Do not offer sweets in exchange for a finished meal.

- Limit amount of television viewing.

- Encourage active play.

- Establish regular family activities, such as walks, ball games, and other outdoor activities.

Rebecca Moran, "Evaluation and Treatment of Childhood Obesity," *American Family Physician* (February 15, 1999), http://www.aafp.org/afp/990215ap/861.html.

"I will praise You, for I am fearfully and wonderfully made."
—Psalm 139:14

I didn't know that the love, the answer I thought was in food, was really, truly, and reliably in Him. A diet certainly couldn't love me. Only God could love me. If only my seven-year-old mind could have realized that.

My first diet ended almost when it started, beginning an endless dieting roller coaster. Diet after diet would start with this angelic-choir Hallelujah moment, followed by this new revelation, "This is the diet. Diet ye in it."

Oftentimes, Mom and I would treat dieting as a buddy project. Mom and I would always start on what day? Monday! Yes, Monday was always the day of the fresh start, the answer. Whenever Mom and I were inspired to go on a diet, we would have one last Sunday blowout, eating all of the "bad food" to get it out of our systems. Then we would be ready to begin our new lives!

Question: Do you believe there are foods that are "good" foods and others that are "bad" foods?

On Monday, there would be commitment and enthusiasm! We'd throw out all the junk food and swear it off forever. We'd institute an exercise program, complete with graph paper and gold stars. Together, we would begin arm circle exercises, bicycle kicks, and sit-ups. Looking back, I find it fitting that these exercises were all movement and no destination. We were moving alright; we just weren't going anywhere. There would also be the measurement, weighing, and counting of ingredients and calories. Mom and I even had our own little notepads, recording our daily menus.

We could usually keep it up for two or three days. Monday was a great start, but every day after it led to our downfall. With each passing day, the Hallelujah choir singing the praises of our new diet was replaced by the songs of our siren stomachs, luring us with praises of forbidden food. Gradually, our written record of "baked potato with pad of butter and carrot sticks" for lunch simply became "potato" (as in chips). Mom and I couldn't bring ourselves to write down the truth, the whole-bag-of-potato-chips truth and nothing-but-potato-chips truth. I couldn't understand why it didn't work. Mom and I did *everything* right. (Everything except pray and trust in God). We had measured everything, except why we were really doing this.

"All the ways of a man are pure in his own eyes,
But the LORD weighs the spirits."
—*Proverbs 16:2*

Our buzzphrase was, "When we get down to our *right* weight." Of course, that must mean we were at our wrong weight. We tried, but eventually, the invitations of chocolate cake, potato chips, and French fries were too strong.

They knew our names and frequently sent us messages. Chocolate cake kept in touch: *Come on, just one bite. Look how sweet I am.* Potato chips were always friendly and social: *Look how crunchy and satisfying I am.* And, of course, the one message that always worked with me with any food whatsoever: *You'll feel better with me. Honest. Come on. You know I still love you.*

And I loved food back. It felt like God to me. Or at least what God should have felt like to me. Food gave me the love, comfort, companionship, parenting, and friendship that I should have found in God. Whenever there was happiness, I turned to food. Whenever there was sorrow, I turned to food. Whenever there was frustration, I turned to food. Whenever there was boredom, uncertainty, pain, any emotion, any feeling in life, I turned to food instead of God.

"But food does not commend us to God,"
—1 Corinthians 8:8

Eventually food turned on me. I thought I was happy with my best friend, but I still felt that I was "wrong."

I was becoming so very aware of exactly how unacceptable I was. It was frequently pointed out to me. Diets were first. Then came the insults, the jokes, the strategies…

"Fatty, Fatty, two by four, can't get through her own front door!"

"She doesn't have to be on our team, does she?"

The old saying is true: "Kids can be cruel." Getting picked last for games, snickering, name-calling, and the shunning were all part of my daily routine.

I once heard about a study of young children. They were asked a question: "If you could choose either an overweight person to be your friend or a person who's missing an arm or a leg, which would you choose?" The kids in the study all chose the missing limbed candidate. Fat, according to the kids then, was unacceptable to be around and befriend.

I came home from school each day and eased my pain with a stack of Oreo cookies, peanut butter and pickle sandwiches, potato chips, and milk. I could feel better with my "true friends."

Insults and jokes from adults were different though. Weren't they supposed to know better? Comments like "You're looking a little pudgy lately" and "Be careful, honey, you don't want to get much fatter now" came from my family and neighbors. During a popular cereal's "can't pinch an inch on me" campaign, they could and did pinch an inch on me. All I wanted was a hug.

I hated one comment most of all. It mainly came from family. In a patronizing, sickly sweet voice, someone would say to me, "You have such a pretty face, if you'd just lose some weight…" There! So my body was what was wrong with me after all! It hurt even more because this comment dangled the hope of beauty, and yet placed the blame on me, a little girl, for not achieving it. It was my fault.

Dressing joined dieting as a new strategy to "fix me." I never really paid much attention to clothes until it was pointed out to me when I was seven years old that I needed to "cover up." I remember my first attempts at dressing in a "slimming" way. I'd wear tight clothes in dark colors (slimming you know) and suck in my stomach. I'd wriggle into tight jeans and try to keep fat rolls from spilling over the waistband. It was both an athletic feat and an "interesting" look. I couldn't breathe very well, but I was successfully "held in." I was also successfully acquiring kidney and bladder infections, due to the restrictive clothes' pressure on my organs. It took my doctor two months to treat these infections. Eventually, I tried another strategy—camouflage. Basically, I wore a tent, anything loose that wouldn't reveal my shape—a big, fat apple.

I became increasingly aware of what my father was and wasn't to me. He was distant, unresponsive, angry, disappointed, and ashamed of me. He wasn't close, involved, happy with me, or proud. I believed that it was entirely my fault because I was an ugly, bad, fat little girl. I needed to be ignored, fixed, and punished. I didn't know that my Heavenly Father felt differently about me. By age ten, I knew only self-imposed hatred, blame, and shame, not my Abba Father's love.

I desperately wanted my dad to notice me. I learned very quickly that one surefire way to do that was by winning awards. When I won something, I wasn't completely worthless or useless. I was productive; I was "earning my keep." I set impossible standards for myself. Try as I might with award after award, I'd eventually disappoint everyone, including myself, proving that I wasn't worth anything after all.

> "In a study by Laliberte, Boland, and Leichner (1999), these three factors represented the hypothesized family climate for eating disorders: perceptions of the family's concern for weight and shape, perceptions of the family's concern for social appearances, and perceptions of the family's emphasis on achievement. The combination of appearance and achievement variables identified in this research describes the perfect family—a family that places great emphasis on appearance, family reputation, family identity, and achievement."
>
> Suzie Csorna, "Familial Relationships and Bulimia," Vanderbilt University Health Psychology Home Page, http://healthpsych.psy .vanderbilt.edu/HealthPsych/families.htm.

My perfect attendance record in school is an excellent example. For three years in a row, I did not missed a single day of school, knowing that I would win a perfect attendance certificate, tangible proof on paper that I was worthwhile. It became a standard I had to maintain because my dad seemed pleased in my performance. Of course, he never said that he was proud of me, but he did lay off the criticisms briefly. So for the next few years, I went to school with colds, sore throats, and influenza. I remember going to school once with a temperature of over 101, sitting at my desk, on the verge of throwing up, yet only thinking of that certificate.

When I reached junior high, I became so sick once I had to stay home. I felt defeated and anxious. My dad, who had never really been sick with so much as a cold, was unsympathetic to my condition. With each passing day I stayed home from school, the tension mounted. Three days at home, according to my dad, was enough. He became upset at my mother for being "such a terrible mother." After three days home, he had enough. He decided he would take me into school to make sure I got there.

On the way to school, he was fuming and I was scared to death, but my 14-year-old mind wanted to know something. We'd never had any father/daughter talks about anything, much less about the existence of a loving relationship, but I got up the nerve to ask him, "Do you still love me?" His answer? "If you do this again, I won't."

His answer proved it. It was my fault. I had to prove myself in order to be loved. I wasn't the cute, good little daughter he should have had. If I could just look right and act right, he'd love me. All I have to do, I decided, is be perfect. That's all.

Nothing worked. I never did achieve perfection. I never got the attention and love I wanted. The scales, numbers, pounds, and inches continued to increase. However, I put on more than weight. As my size increased, so did my shame, defeat, and failure. I didn't know that God already loved me as is. I wasn't aware that God would even care about any of this.

I was, after all, just a fat girl.

"*Then you shall feed;*
On her sides shall you be carried,
And be dandled on her knees.
As one whom his mother comforts,
So I will comfort you"
—*Isaiah 66:12—13*

A **Prayer** to Rise

Father, I come to You in the name of Jesus, asking for Your help in my life. Thank You for knowing and loving me completely. You know all of the struggles I'm facing concerning food. I confess that I have turned to food to be my source of love, comfort, and joy when I should be turning to You instead. I ask for forgiveness for that. Be Lord and Savior over my body and life.

Father, I ask for You to help me with my attitudes, choices, and behaviors toward food. Where I have incorrect, unhealthy approaches, I ask, Lord, for You to give me guidance and wisdom as to how and what I am supposed to eat in order to be Your healthy creation.

In the name and by the blood of Jesus, I cast down wrong ways of thinking and feeling about myself, whether they are from my childhood or more recent days. I ask for forgiveness in these matters, involving each person concerned. Help me to learn Your love and Your ways, how to be Your daughter, in spirit, soul, and body, so that I may love and glorify You and be who You created me to be. I ask all of this in Jesus's name. Amen.

Journaling Section

To Help You **Work Through** Your Thoughts

Name three things (excluding your size, appearance, or weight) that are precious and loveable about you. (**Isaiah 43:4**)

- my compassion
- my creativity
- my desire to keep growing

How does food make you feel? What are your emotions when you eat?

- like I am being hugged inside out, love being poured into me.
- pleasure till the point of sickness

Complete these statements concerning what and how you eat and feel.

When I feel stressed, I eat (list foods)

- chocolate
- granola bars
- pie
- buttered bread

And I feel (list emotions)

- fraction of relief
- sickness
- hatred
- depressed

After eating I feel (list emotions)

What is one harmful thing you learned from being on a diet as a child? How can you let God heal that for you now?

- I was still growing.
- It never works - back fires

- releasing it's control on me

Name three things about yourself that, according to **Psalm 139:14**, makes you "fearfully and wonderfully made"?

- complexity
- made in God's image
- made with purpose

Make a list of what you consider to be good or safe foods and what you consider to be bad or dangerous foods. Explain why you see them that way.

Good	Bad
• fruit	• chocolate
• vegetables	• cake
• oats	• pie
• un salted nuts	• muffins
• boiled unsalted egg	• breads?
• water	• cereal
• healthy not un natural	• cookies
	• red meat
	• milk
	• perservatives
	salts, fats, Un natural

Why have you gone on a diet? What's been your motive for dieting/losing weight? Read **Proverbs 16:2**. How do you think God sees your plan? What can you do to include God in a healthy plan now?

• get peoples attention that I'm worth being around
• to have control over how I look which will lead to what people will talk about.

What are potential risks in dieting? What have you gone through healthwise that has affected your health/life personally? ① • Obsessing over weight

② • bulimia

• binging

• cutting myself

• burning myself

• hitting myself

• drug & alcohol addiction

Matthew 6:25 suggests that life is more important than food. List what is more important than food to you.

• Relationships with people

• future career

• God

• family

What do you think God wants for your health and life?

_____

_____

_____

_____

_____

_____

_____

How do you feel about trusting God? Trusting others? How do you think these feelings affect your relationship toward food and your eating patterns?

_____

_____

_____

_____

_____

_____

_____

_____

_____

Read **Isaiah 66:12–13**, then complete the following statements:

God can comfort me in the following ways:

_____

_____

_____

_____

_____

_____

I would like to be comforted in the following ways:

_____

_____

_____

_____

_____

_____

Scriptures to Consider

Job 33:29–30   Proverbs 16:2
Isaiah 43:4   Matthew 6:25
1 Corinthians 8:8   Isaiah 66:12–3
Psalm 139:14

Chapter Two

Famine

Famine (Little Girl Decided)

Famine aged her
with the promise of a childhood forever,
safety forever
perfect forever,
never good enough
she was,
"Just make me a stick figure,
Just make me disappear,
I must
I must
I must be as small as dust"
Famine would fix everything,
make everything all right.
Smaller
just take up
less space
less room
a tomb preserving a little girl.
She wouldn't have to grow up
the little girl told herself.
"Don't want anything
Don't be anything,
Just be small,
Nothing,

No trouble
at all,"
Concentration camp minefield—she learned,
"My mind doesn't mind
anymore,
My mind isn't mine
Anymore."
She learned from her invisible corset,
cinching her
waist,
"I can't breathe anymore,
I can't think, I can't feel
anymore,
I'm only real
the more
I can feel my bones"
Little girl decided
Beauty
Duty
it was to take up,
just take up
less space
less room,
"That's what I want to be when I grow up—
Less"
Scary hell
Don't tell her
ever
She might
have to grow up,
"Please God,

Don't let me grow up,"
the growling of her stomach
The Little Girl's Amen,
It answered the whisper
Approval
She
was wrong,
But
She would fix that.
Famine
"I must
I must
I must be as small as dust."

Diet and defeat, attempts and failure had become my way of life. That is, until one day, when diet became *victory* for me. And little by little, attempt by attempt, pound by pound, inch by inch, I succeeded at cutting away the excess weight. But more than that, I found control, victory, accomplishment, worth, and perfection.

Question: Do you feel you must be perfect at everything you do?

I took control. "All right," I said to myself, "if I can't have the love, the worthiness, the me that I want, I'll make it on my own." Control became the name of the game now. Even though I thought it was the beginning of my promised land, this was when the real danger, the real wilderness began.

Question: Do you feel in control of your life when you control your food and weight?

The summer after my senior year of high school became my "put up or shut up" summer. As I prepared for college, I had a lot to prove—to myself, to my jeering classmates, to the boys who had *not* been asking me out. I had to prove that I was a worthwhile, beautiful girl. During my entire adolescence, I had been the fat girl, the "good friend," the funny sidekick to the beautiful girls. But that would all change *this* summer.

So I started another diet. At 18, I'd had years of failure at diet and exercise programs. I don't know what was so different this time, except that this time I was *determined*—determined to reinvent myself for my new life at college.

> "More than half of teenaged girls are, or think they should be, on diets. They want to lose all or some of the 40 pounds that females naturally gain between 8 and 14. About 3 percent of these teens go too far, becoming anorexic or bulimic."
> ANRED, "Statistics: How Many People Have Eating Disorders?" http://www.anred.com/stats.html. Used with permission.

I started looking for role models I could pattern myself after. I chose Audrey Hepburn for her thin, delicate beauty. I chose Madonna to be my fitness and female empowerment guide. She was a beautiful, lean, muscular version of what I'd deemed a woman "having it all" was like. I thought they had perfect lives, and mine would be perfect too if I could be as beautiful as they were. I coveted who these women were. So much for the "no other gods" commandment. I was breaking that one daily as I looked to these feminine idols for inspiration instead of to God to be my inspiration. I pursued my own idol of perfect, thin beauty and self-obsession.

Question: Do you compare yourself with other girls and women regarding your physical appearance?

Idols are still around for the coveting and worshiping. That hasn't changed. I found my idols in Hollywood.

In Hollywood, there is a trend for actresses to be an unusually thin size. It seems to be a competitive "who's the thinnest one of them all" scenario, pressuring actresses to slim down to not just a size 8 or 6 dress, but to even go as low as a size 0.

Size 0! Since actresses sell, in part, their physical appearance, unwillingness or inability to whittle down to a tiny size automatically translates into being "less marketable" and "difficult." They can lose anything from their popularity to actual work in film and television.

Take for instance, the female cast of the television show *Friends*. When the show began ten years ago, the actresses were at more normal, healthy weights. However, the more popular the show became, the more weight the cast lost. Media controversy swirled around their thinning bodies. Whether or not they were anorexic or bulimic, it still sent a dangerous, confusing message: The thinner you are, the more successful you will be in your life and career.

I know beyond a shadow of a doubt that if I had watched the series at 19, the thin female cast members would have been my personal standard of what women should look like and be: a size 0 in all of its glory.

We have had somewhat of a turn in the media's present standard. People like the actress Kate Winslet, entertainer Beyonce Knowles, and the full-figure model Emme have presented themselves as being beautiful, talented, real women who aren't a size 0. Jennifer Lopez (with her much-discussed derriere) is also a positive role model for healthy self-image, living proof that the female shape and female curves are not necessarily something to lose. Women do come in *all* shapes and sizes.

Let me encourage any young girl or woman out there right now, *you* are the standard, not the images you see on TV and film. They are illusions. Even the famous, thin models on magazine covers don't look like that naturally. They are given stylists, makeup and hair designers, great lighting, and airbrush effects to achieve their "perfect" look. It's a product, not a person.

Be careful in choosing your role models and goals. Look to God's tried and true Word, not Hollywood, to find your worth.

"I have chosen you and have not cast you away."
—*Isaiah 41:9*

Question: Do you feel you are worthy of love only when you are thin or look a certain way?

Unfortunately, I bought the wrong product; I bought the lie. With my role models in place and my mind made up, I plowed straight ahead with my goals. I drank diet drinks that tasted like chocolate-flavored chalk. I started exercising on a stationary bike, a real bike, and a mini trampoline. The exercise sped up my success. I started losing weight and keeping it off! I felt exhilaration and power. I started exercising an hour every day, pedaling on my bikes or jumping up and down on the trampoline to music in my family's basement.

For the first time in my life, people appreciated my body, my looks. People now referred to me as "tiny" and "cute." People were now coming up to me, saying things like, "Keep it up," "Keep doing what you're doing," and (with a happy smile on their face, of course) "You've lost weight!" I'd had years of people complimenting me for my talent, mind, good personality, and sense of humor, but these new compliments were *intoxicating!* I realized the truth of the statement: "Nothing tastes as good as thin feels." For me, being thinner qualified me to be loved and accepted by others.

Guys were now approving of me, flirting with me. They now hugged, touched me—they even picked me up and carried me around. I was thrilled. My whole life, I'd not been held like this, picked up like this, not even by my own father. And now guys were physically and emotionally whisking me off my feet.

I also loved the fact that I could wear clothes that were stylish, whose design wasn't to camouflage, to hide, to deny "unsightly" lumps, bumps, rolls. I could go in and try on a size six dress and find it too big for me! Yesss! I could step on a scale, fully dressed, including shoes and a coat, and only register 120 pounds.

Each comment, lost pound, and lost inch gave me more of an incentive. As I lost weight, I found myself always in need of a new goal. If 115 pounds looked this great on me, why stop there? I eventually became convinced that death—at least the look of starvation—was beautiful. I was envying the "beauty," the look of the malnourished, the tortured—even those in concentration camps. I now went beyond looking to Audrey Hepburn and Madonna as role models and influences. They were now competition for me. If I could be thinner than these women, then I'd be better than they were as well.

Ah, at long last, control over *something* in my life. I couldn't control who loved me or what was going on in my family, but I could control *this*! I could control my body! And soon this control did turn into something I'd hungered for, craved my entire life: power, power in the beauty, the newfound thin beauty I was discovering. College would be a new beginning for sure, I thought. I was the Sheryle I always thought I wanted to be.

Competition grew between me and any thin girl or woman. Mirror, mirror: I had to be the thinnest one of them all. It was life or death importance, anything less than that was unacceptable. Gaining any weight whatsoever meant failure, simple as that.

Question: Do you feel like you are a failure if you gain weight?

So to keep going on my quest for perfection, a thin body deserving of love and approval, I increased the amount of exercise and decreased what I ate. I went from bike pedaling or trampoline jumping one hour to two hours now. From there, I pushed myself to three and four hours of exercise every morning. During this time, I decreased my calories from 1,500 to 1,200 to 1,000.

It still wasn't good enough. I *had* to exercise six hours a day every day on 800 calories. I made it a constant goal to drop 100 calories after a certain period of time, after I'd achieved a certain loss in pounds or inches. And as I studied myself more and more in the mirror, I felt that the weight, the fat, wasn't coming off quickly enough.

What I didn't realize at the time was that my eyes and mind were incapable of seeing anything but a distorted image. Each time I looked at myself in the mirror, all I saw was a fat baby picture of me with fat arms, fat legs, and double chin. I'd spent most of my young life being that photograph. I'd do whatever was needed to make sure that it wasn't the case now.

Diary Entry (March 22, 1991)

Got up, sit-ups, weights… worked on the trampoline for 2 hours, 50 minutes—great—did extra sit-ups. Weighed myself—found out I weigh 115 pounds! Wow!!! I can't believe it! All of the exercise and dieting is paying off—

I want to lose more weight, though. Before history class, I saw Stacy, and she said I looked different—thinner. Yeah!

"A sound heart is life to the body,
But envy is rottenness to the bones."
—Proverbs 14:30

My 120 pounds became 115, which then dropped down to 110. I could feel my hip bones, and it was uncomfortable for me to sit in chairs. But I was succeeding. That's all that mattered. And besides, I wouldn't go *too* far. I'd stop when I was satisfied. Yeah, when I was at my "right" weight, then I'd stop. After all, I was in control.

Soon 110 pounds gave way to 100 pounds. I was great. I was fine. I had to wear two or three layers of clothing all of the time just to keep warm, but it was a small price to pay, right?

Then the comments started to change. Instead of the usual, "You look great," I started getting more questions like, "Are you okay?" "You've lost weight" was now said with a concerned look and worried tone, not a smile. I started getting the question, "Are you eating?" A former high school classmate who had been anorexic became concerned. Within a span of four months, she approached me three times and asked me if I was anorexic. I defensively denied it each time. She terrified and infuriated me. Did any of these people asking these dreaded questions understand that they were trying to wreck everything I'd been striving to accomplish? I made up my mind. They were my enemy. They were trying to stop my success, my victory. But I wouldn't let them. I intended to keep going.

One hundred pounds dropped to 90 pounds. By this time, I wasn't feeling so hot at all. I was constantly freezing, now wearing three to four layers of clothing, despite the fact that it was a hot and humid mid-July. I was "feeling worse," but believing that I was "looking better." At 90 pounds, my skin was crepe paper and just hung off from my bones. It didn't have enough muscle tone or fat to support any kind of shape. Of course, I saw this as "fat flab." I started losing hair in patches at my temples. My teeth were thinning, the enamel wasting away. I could count all of my ribs. I still wasn't thin enough; it wasn't good enough. I looked at myself and all I saw was the fat girl: disgusting, unworthy, not perfect or lovable. You know what that meant—more exercise (six plus hours a day) and less food (600 or less calories a day).

I was determined to reach my perfect weight goal of 80 pounds. At this point, I felt shame. Guilt increased every time someone questioned me. I was ashamed. I knew that what I was doing was wrong, but I still kept going. I had to. Progress—just a few more pounds, then I'll be done. So I'd continue every morning: six hours of boot camp torture on little or no food or water. I had gotten to the point where I feared drinking water would make me fat.

Question: Do you take actions to get and keep yourself thin at all costs?

Every morning, my heart and pulse would pound and race. I could feel throbbing from veins that were sticking out on the backs of my knees and the crooks of my elbows. Every morning, I would stand up, shaky, dizzy already, only to then have everything go black. And then, I'd wake up, lying on the floor.

I was scared now, not only for my health, but scared of the danger of being discovered. What if I did this in front of someone? You see, these daily blackout sessions always happened during my exercise routine at midnight. I started exercising at midnight because I could be alone for my required six-hour exercise punishment. I was afraid of what people—especially my family—would think if I collapsed in front of them.

Mom frequently told me, "When you lie down to sleep, I'm afraid you'll never wake up." She'd also pick up library books on anorexia and read me the symptoms, commenting on things like the hair loss, the father issues, the obsession with not eating, etc. It was during this time, desperate to keep control of the situation, I did what I call "mock eating," where I made it look like I'd eaten more than I did. I'd put some food on a plate and "disturb it" enough. It was all designed to make her believe that I was eating. This thought scared me too.

My parents began threatening me with hospitalization. I only worried that they threatened to take my *control* away.

I was hiding, feeling nothing but fear and shame. I must protect this! I must! At this point, I became obsessed with self-protection, self-preservation. Funny, huh? I was basically near death, and yet I saw self-preservation as maintaining control.

Question: Do you hide your behaviors when it comes to food, weight, and body issues?

I was feeling more and more uncomfortable now. At 80 pounds, I'd gotten to the point where it was physically uncomfortable—painful for me to even lie down or sit. I had no energy to keep going, but I couldn't rest. My hip bones, spine, and tailbone stuck out so much I could feel a stabbing pain whenever

I tried to get comfortable. I couldn't get rest. Sleeping became impossible.

"My heart throbs, my strength fails me;
And the light of my eyes, even that has gone from me.
For I hope in you, O LORD; You will answer,
O Lord my God." —Psalm 38:10, 15 NASB

I was tired physically, emotionally, spiritually. I just existed, going through the motions each day. I didn't want to be here anymore. At 19 years 8 months, I daily prayed, "God, just let me die. Don't let me make it to age 20." I know it's because of God's love for me that I'm still here. I thank God He didn't answer those prayers the way I wanted. I'm alive. I should have been dead more times than I survived. There but for the grace of God. . . .

Question: Do you ever have thoughts of wanting to die?

I remember priding myself whenever I heard about other anorexics dying at heavier weights than I was at. To me, that symbolized my strength. Yeah, I was so much stronger, better than they were. See, they were the ones who had the problem. They couldn't handle it. I could. How wrong I was. It was God who was strong, not me. It was God who was still keeping me alive.

Although I was reaching my goals, I still felt wrong, empty, and a failure. I was constantly afraid—afraid to eat, to live, to die, to move, to stand. I was afraid of people, of having them stare at me, afraid that they would somehow know what was going on. I worried that they had this crazy idea that I was dying. They didn't see my victory, my goals being set and achieved.

Question: Do you often feel afraid and ashamed of your eating behavior?

One of my goals was fitting into a bridesmaid dress for my cousin's wedding. She asked me in March to be a bridesmaid in her summer wedding. At that time, I weighed around 115–120 pounds, which translated into a size 9/10 dress.

By June, I was about 95–100 pounds and the dress swallowed me. I felt my accomplishment as the seamstress cinched in the sides of the waist. Yes, I was getting smaller. My cousin could only look at my mother in stunned, horrified disbelief. But, hey, I was successful!

Question: Do people around you (family and friends) make comments about your weight loss or appearance?

I really started obsessing the two weeks prior to the wedding. Looking back on my diary entries, I wrote a repetitive string of comments like "I'm not going to eat today or tomorrow" and "I can't blow it now. I'm so close." I was desperate to convince my mother that I was just "slimming down" for a special occasion. To prove myself, I asked for the two of us to draw up a written agreement. In it we "agreed" that 90 pounds would be acceptable once the wedding was over. In the meantime, I continued days straight without eating, accompanied by hours of excessive exercise, 2,000–4,000 sit-ups a day—insanity.

The August wedding eventually came and proved to be both anticlimactic and tense. The buildup, the hype, the "end-all, be-all" quality I had attached to it was replaced with a disappointing reality. At 82 pounds, I tried on the dress and discovered that's all it was—just a dress. Yes, it was hanging on me, but it didn't really mean anything anymore. I was too exhausted for it to mean anything to me. I had to pin the sides of the dress with safety pins. It was hanging from my 20-inch waist (18 inches, if I held in my breath).

Despite the fact that I was freezing, I was determined to wear this girly pink southern belle extravaganza off the shoulder. Mom, however, felt differently and with a look of disgust on her face, kept pushing up the shoulders on the dress. It was more than just a mother/daughter appropriate dressing situation here. She was trying to cover up her grotesque daughter with her grotesque collarbones and her grotesque shoulder blades. I was an embarrassment, something to be ashamed of, repulsed by—again.

All day, I got double takes and felt constant stares. Family and guests at the wedding, one by one, stared just a little too long, making me uncomfortable. Here I was, my whole life craving attention, but not this! People stammered things like, "Sheryle, you look...pretty" and "My, you're thin. I didn't recognize you." They obviously felt uncomfortable saying it. A guy cousin of mine said something like, "Man, you're thin [two beats of awkward silence], but...you...you look...good." He said it to me like I was in danger of dying right there.

It was a long day. I focused most of my concentration on just staying vertical and not fainting. I had accomplished my goal; I was skinny for this wedding. I was just too exhausted and hollow to enjoy it.

Question: Do you consider yourself to be fat even when people comment on how thin you are?

My mother held me to our pact when the wedding was over. I'd dress for my "weigh in," starting off with my workout clothes, a leotard, or a one-piece number of some sort. I'd then put on my long johns over that, with a T-shirt, plus exercise pants and the matching shirt. This helped a lot in keeping me a little bit warmer. I then added a large flannel shirt and some baggy jeans—of course, any jeans at this point were baggy. I was wearing jeans that I wore when I was 12 years old. I was 19 now, and they were enormous on me. I wore two pairs of socks to top it all off.

I'd approach Mom, confident in my armor and I'd step on the scale. Because I weighed myself several times a day, I knew I should only register 80–85 pounds. But with all of this, I felt triumphant as I watched the needle on the scale flicker to the 98-pound mark—a "safe" number for my family to see.

I was "safe" once again, even though I was tired all of the time. At least I was living "in control." I started feeling really guilty, especially when I prayed. I didn't know what God thought of me now. Did He still love me? You see, something different started happening. I started changing once again. And this time, I definitely had no control over what was happening.

Question: Do you feel that God loves you as you are *right now?*

A **Prayer** to Rise

Father, I come to You in the name of Jesus, asking for help in my life. I thank You that You are the God of all hope and miracles. I ask for both hope and miracles now in Jesus's name. As much as I don't want to admit it, I am anorexic and need Your healing touch upon me. I confess I have lived in denial, lying to You, to myself, and to others about what is going on with me. I have hurt myself and others, and I ask for Your forgiveness for that.

Lord, You know I'm scared, not only of gaining weight and of losing control, but of so many other things as well. I ask for Your help; I ask for Your deliverance. I don't want to keep going this way. Please heal me and give me courage to change.

I confess I've made weight, size, and image into idols to worship instead of focusing on You as my only God. I ask You to forgive me and help me to love and worship You in spirit and in truth (**John 4:24**).

Father, I feel hopeless, unworthy, ugly, and unlovable right now. I ask for You to love me and help me see my value through Your eyes, beyond my weight and how I look. I am hurting right now, and I ask for Your healing upon me.

I don't feel like I am Your beautiful, created, chosen daughter right now. Please change that. Change me with Your healing love. In Jesus's name, I pray. Amen.

Journaling Section

To Help You **Work Through** Your Thoughts

Why would losing weight make you better? What do you think would change for the better if you were thinner?

_____

_____

_____

_____

_____

_____

How do you feel when you control your food weight and appearance? How do you feel when you are not in control?

_____

_____

_____

_____

_____

_____

_____

List girls or women you compare yourself with or especially admire. List what it is that you think they have that you don't possess. Why do you want these traits?

_____

_____

_____

_____

_____

_____

Now, using the previous exercise, list what you have that they don't have (only positive things you like about yourself). Explain why you like those traits.

Physical Appearance

God gave me _____ that

(name) _____ doesn't have. I like my

_____ because _____

_____

Personality and Talents

God gave me _____ that

(name) _____ doesn't have. I like my

_____ because _____

_____

What form(s) of exercise do you participate in and why do you exercise?

_____

_____

_____

_____

_____

What can you do to incorporate God into your exercise plan?

_____

_____

_____

_____

_____

What are ways God can make exercise more healthy and fun for you?

_____

_____

_____

_____

Isaiah 41:9 states that God has chosen and not rejected you. How do you feel about that statement?

_____

_____

_____

_____

_____

_____

_____

Describe an experience in which you felt rejected. Who was it that made you feel that way? How did you respond? How do you feel about it today?

_____

_____

_____

_____

_____

_____

_____

_____

Describe an experience in which you felt chosen. Who was it that made you feel that way? How did you respond? How do you feel about it today?

_____

_____

_____

_____

_____

_____

Proverbs 14:30 states that envy rots the bones. What does that mean to you? Of whom are you envious? What could you do, through God's help, to change those feelings?

_____

_____

_____

_____

_____

_____

_____

_____

According to **Psalm 38:10, 15 (NASB, NRSV, or NIV)**, the Lord will answer. Name an instance in the past in which God has answered your prayer.

_____

_____

_____

_____

_____

_____

Based on **Psalm 38:10, 15**, write God a prayer you want answered now. Then listen carefully for His answer.

_____

_____

_____

_____

_____

_____

_____

_____

_____

_____

_____

List below what you believe to be your perfect weight and size.

Perfect weight: _____   Bust: _____

Perfect dress size: _____   Waist: _____

Height: _____   Hips: _____

The table below compares average women in the US with Barbie dolls and department store mannequins. It's not encouraging.

	Average Woman	Barbie	Store Mannequin
Height	5' 4"	6' 0"	6' 0"
Weight	145 lb.	101 lb.	Not available
Dress size	11–14	4	6
Bust	36–37"	39"	34"
Waist	29–31"	19"	23"
Hips	40–42"	33"	34"

Health magazine (September 1997); and NEDIC, a Canadian eating disorders advocacy group, as cited in ANRED, "Statistics: How Many People Have Eating Disorders?" http://www.anred.com/stats.html. Used with permission.

After reviewing the table, how do you feel about the statistics given compared with your information? What do you think of the chart?

_____

_____

_____

_____

_____

_____

_____

List a time when someone made a comment about your appearance. What was it? How did it make you feel then? How does it make you feel now?

_____

_____

_____

_____

_____

_____

_____

_____

_____

Have you ever made a comment about someone else's appearance? What did you say? How did you feel after you said it?

_____

_____

_____

_____

_____

_____

Do you consider yourself to be fat right now? Why or why not?

_____

_____

_____

_____

_____

_____

_____

_____

_____

Aside from any food, weight, or body issues, what in life brings you joy, happiness, or excitement?

_____

_____

_____

_____

_____

_____

_____

Do you feel that God loves you as you are *right now*? Why or why not?

_____

_____

_____

_____

_____

_____

_____

Scriptures to Consider

Isaiah 41:9 **Psalm 38:10, 15**

Personality Characteristics of Individuals with Anorexia Nervosa

- Perfectionists
- Conflict avoidant
- Emotionally and sexually inhibited
- Compliant
- Approval seeking
- Excessively dependent
- Socially anxious
- Fearful of spontaneity
- Reluctant to take risks
- Practices food rituals

Characteristics of Families of Persons with Anorexia Nervosa

- Enmeshed, overprotective, conflict avoiding
- Unresponsive to patient's self-expressions
- Discourage independence
- Patient overly dependent on parents
- Parents may urge young daughters to lose weight

Adapted from Ohio State University FactSheet (July 4, 2003), "Eating Disorders Awareness: Emotional Issues Involved with Eating Disorders," http://ohioline.osu.edu/ed-fact/1005.html.

If You Have Anorexia Nervosa

- Don't diet. Never ever. Instead design a meal plan that gives your body all the nutrition it needs for health and growth. Also get 30 to 60 minutes of exercise or physical activity three to five days a week. More than that is too much.
- Ask someone you trust for an honest, objective opinion of your weight. If they say you are normal weight or thin, believe them.
- When you start to get overwhelmed by "feeling fat," push beyond the anxiety and ask yourself what you are really afraid of. Then take steps to deal with the threat if it is real or dismiss it if it is not real.

ANRED, "Self-Help Tips," http://www.anred.com/slf_hlp.html. Used with permission.

Chapter Three

Prison

Prison (Now You've Done It)

A prison
made out of every fork tine,
Her prison
Her answer
She called it
"Mine,"
Each fork full,
Prison,
The little girl sent herself
there,
Now
you've done it,
Now
you've eaten it,
Now
What's left?
Get rid of it!
She felt that God left her anyway
Holding onto the fork,
the little girl didn't know
where else to go
other than to prison,
She ate
She did the unforgivable,

Now
The little girl had to get
control,
Bad
Bad
Bad,
Punish her,
Because eating had the meaning
of being
fat,
unacceptable.

There comes a point when you just get so hungry, you'll do anything to eat.

For the longest time, I'd prided myself on becoming this special creature. I'd convinced myself that I was different; I didn't need to eat like other people did.

I'd managed to make it through this anorexic summer by dealing with things "my way." I felt it was necessary for me to get away from my parents, from their suspicious eyes and dangerous threats. I thought to myself every day that summer, "I just have to make it to September, and then I'll be free. I just need to get out of here." Moving out was becoming increasingly important as I began to give in to the occasional binge, which was causing me to panic.

Diary Entry (August 23, 1991)

I'm feeling pretty low today—I got up and weighed myself at 85 pounds. Then I ate a lot. I had eight slices of white bread with peanut butter, two or three with maple syrup, two bananas, one peach, two cucumbers, green beans, two peanut butter micro diet bars, one chocolate bar, blueberry and apple pie filling, All Bran, Grape Nuts, Cream of Wheat all mixed with honey—it's early evening now and I'm up to 92–93 pounds. I rode my bike for an hour and only did 1,000 sit-ups—no weights—already feel guilty about that. I feel awful. My stomach and back hurt. I should not have eaten today, but at least I'm now sick of food. I should have Mom off my case now. She's seen me eat, and I'm hoping to keep her at bay. I resent Mom right now. I know it was me who ate the food, but she's making the situation tense, making me feel obligated to eat, and then I can't stop. I'm hoping the exercise I did today will burn off this weight.

Question: Are you angry with anyone, especially when they mention your eating habits and weight?

By the end of the summer, Mom's pressure to eat was increasing. She made more hospitalization threats, telling me I was crazy. Anger welled up in me when she'd say things like that. I wanted to lash out at her, to hurt her back by screaming at her, "You're what is wrong with me! The fact that I have to do this for you to pay attention to me, the fact that I have to work to earn your love and attention—that's what's wrong with me!" However, I just kept quiet, strengthening my resolve and waiting until glorious September when I would be free.

College finally came. I felt hope at the thought of freedom on my own terms. Things would be different. Now I could concentrate and be happy. I moved into an apartment with two roommates. Miraculously, I was able to be a functioning student, keep good grades, and regularly attend my classes. I kept up the "okay" facade.

However, I couldn't stop the changes going on in my body. It started out with a shift in my thinking. I found myself more obsessed and tortured by food. Suddenly I wanted food right now! And after all, I was 80 pounds. I could afford a little something to eat, right?

I was nervous. This went against everything I'd been working for. Do something on my forbidden list? Put weight on instead of taking it off? I would move closer to the fat, unacceptable me that I was trying so hard not to be. But my hunger went beyond a growling stomach. True starvation will make you entertain thoughts you wouldn't dare think otherwise.

Question: Is food constantly on your mind?

Nothing else mattered anymore. Everything else was fuzzy around me: right and wrong, other people, God, consequences. Just food mattered. But things were different now. Innocence toward food was gone. I couldn't simply "just eat" again. You can't go back once you've been down my road. It's never again quite as simple as "just eat."

I suddenly became aware of all the food around me: food that I had sworn off, food I'd forbidden. When alone in our apartment, I was tortured by my roommates' food. I was hungry, and I was tempted: *Come on, just this once. Your roommates will never miss this food. They'll never know it's gone. Besides, it's just this once, and then you'll get back on track.*

I'd always believed that stealing was wrong—a "thou shalt not." Right? But I was so hungry, right and wrong didn't matter.

Question: Do you want to eat but feel you don't deserve food?

When I began eating (stealing) my roommates' food, I felt warring emotions. Feasting on boxes of rice and crackers, granola bars, fistfuls of cereals, and ice cream bars felt wonderful. But I began to panic. Where would all of this show up on me? My straight hips? My 20-inch waist? My hollow cheekbones? I wanted to protect the product of my hard work. Still, I couldn't stop eating. Every time, I repeated my new vow, "I'll do this just one time." One time became always.

Question: Do you binge on food whenever you experience negative feelings?

"For what I am doing, I do not understand.
For what I will to do, that I do not practice;
but what I hate, that I do."
—Romans 7:15

After each feast, I felt exhaustion, guilt, shame, and pain. My body wasn't able to deal with this violent attack of food. I was literally stuffed with food. My stomach was extremely distended. I looked like a pregnant, malnourished refugee. My stomach was rock hard and stretched beyond its limits. I was uncomfortable standing, sitting, walking, and breathing. I paced back and forth in my apartment, trying to get comfortable. I hated myself and felt like the most horrible, disgusting person in the world. Who would want and love me now? What boy? What man? I even started to question—What God?

I moved into a new eating disorder. Every day, I'd start out weighing 80-something pounds. I would be tempted, gorge, panic, binge, and weigh myself. Each time, I would shoot back up to 90 pounds again. My urgent prayer became, "Oh God, no, help me. You know I can't weigh this."

I didn't realize until years later that my supposed daily "weight gain" really wasn't a weight gain at all. There was no way for my body to absorb all of those thousands of calories in that short time. My immediate "weight gains" only reflected the massive volume of food and water I was consuming. It stands to reason that when a person drinks anything whatsoever, the body will immediately absorb it. It will then register on the scale as well. Realistically, there was no way I could put on ten pounds in one hour.

I also didn't realize my mind was set in a destructive pattern of bingeing and purging, medically known as bulimia. All I knew was that the scale said 90 pounds. I would cry myself to sleep by begging God not to hate me and to make my life stop. I didn't want to live anymore.

"Four out of one hundred college-aged women have bulimia. About 50 percent of people who have been anorexic develop bulimia or bulimic patterns."
ANRED, "Statistics: How Many People Have Eating Disorders?"
http://www.anred.com/stats.html. Used with permission.

It's amazing how things sneak up on you. For years now I'd been in denial about my issues with food and weight. First, I convinced myself that I could hide my weight with clothing and sheer will. Then, I was in denial about being too thin, convincing myself that I could cover that, too. And now, here I was, trying to convince myself that this third eating disorder, bulimia, wasn't a reality. It was a "just this one time" thing.

"Whoever has no rule over his own spirit
Is like a city broken down, without walls."
—Proverbs 25:28

I started each day with good intentions, but my cravings and my body were turning on me. Temptation was too strong now. I was rehooked on the high that food brought. I'd been so long without it, and it brought me such comfort. Food became my answer again. I hadn't really grown up. Having an eating disorder suspended me as a little girl with no curves, no menstrual cycle (which I had not had for six months), and no sexuality.

Bulimia was making all the decisions now. I didn't have the control to decide my "right weight" anymore. It was deciding me. It became my cruel, demanding god. It was all I ever thought about.

"Is not life more than food?"
—Jesus, in Matthew 6:25

A **Prayer** to Rise

Father, I come to You in the name of Jesus, asking for help in my life. Thank You, Lord, that You are a God with whom nothing is impossible (Luke 1:37). Lord, right now in my life, things seem impossible and unbearable. I ask for help as I recognize my behavior as being that of bulimia. I confess that I am suffering from this and need Your divine help to intervene. I admit I cannot make any change; I cannot improve my life by myself. I need Your help.

Lord, You know the extremes I've experienced through bingeing and purging. You know the toll it has taken on me spiritually, emotionally, and physically. It has consumed my life in an unhealthy way. I ask for forgiveness, and I turn to You to fill any void, any weakness I have with more of You and Your love.

Lord, I feel trapped, and I ask You to free me from this prison. I pray for Your help and healing upon my emotions. I need You to set me free. Guide me through these difficulties to Your loving promises and to Your divine help in every area of my life. I ask this in Jesus's name. Amen.

Journaling Section

To Help You **Work Through** Your Thoughts

What about your current life makes you feel like you're in prison? How do you see God setting you free from that prison?

_____

_____

_____

_____

_____

_____

Are you angry with anyone, especially when they mention anything concerning your eating habits and weight? What have they said? What's been your reaction?

_____

_____

_____

_____

_____

_____

What problems exist in your life now that cause you to turn to food and/or dieting to solve? How could you turn to God instead?

_____

_____

_____

_____

_____

_____

What are your thoughts concerning food?

_____

_____

_____

_____

Do you want to eat, but feel you don't deserve food? If so, why do you feel that way?

_____

_____

_____

_____

How does **Romans 7:15** relate to your life and circumstances when it comes to food? What do you see as being the answer?

_____

_____

_____

_____

_____

_____

_____

Who or what makes you feel safe? How do you think God could make you feel safe? What steps could you take right now to make that happen?

_____

_____

_____

_____

_____

_____

_____

How do you feel about your level of self-control? What does **Proverbs 25:28** mean to you?

_____

_____

_____

_____

_____

_____

_____

_____

_____

Scriptures to Consider

Romans 7:15	**Proverbs 25:28**
Isaiah 43:4	**Matthew 6:25**

Personality Characteristics of Individuals with Bulimia

- Unstable moods, thought patterns, behavior, and self-images
- Cannot stand to be alone
- Demand constant attention
- Difficulty controlling impulsive behavior
- Secretive behavior

Indications of Bulimia, Anorexia Nervosa, and Binge Eating Disorders

- Inability to soothe oneself or to empathize with others
- Need for admiration
- Hypersensitivity to criticism or defeat
- Frequently experience depression
- Depression common in families
- Low amounts of neurotransmitters
- Low amounts of tryptophan

Characteristics Noted in Families of Persons with Bulimia

- Critical and detached parents
- Characterized by hostile enmeshment
- Nonnurturing
- Emotionally unresponsive
- Parent possibly obese, experiencing an eating disorder, or overweight during childhood

Adapted from Ohio State University FactSheet, http://ohioline.osu.edu/ed-fact/1005.html. Used with permission.

If You Have Bulimia Nervosa
or Binge Eating Disorder

- Don't let yourself get too hungry, too angry, too frustrated, too lonely, too tired, or too bored. All these states are powerful binge triggers. Watch for them, and when they first appear, deal with them in a healthy manner instead of letting the tension build until bingeing and purging become the conceivable release.
- Stay comfortably busy and avoid unstructured time. Empty time is too easily filled with binge food.
- Make sure that every day you touch base with friends and loved ones. Enjoy being with them. It sounds corny, but hugs really are healing.
- Take control of your life. Make choices thoughtfully and deliberately. Make your living situation safe and comfortable.
- Every day do something fun, something relaxing, something energizing.
- Monitor your self-talk. Challenge self-critical nagging. Deliberately choose to change the subject and count your blessings when you fall into negative thoughts about yourself, your appearance, your abilities, and your accomplishments.
- Keep tabs on your feelings. Several times a day ask yourself how you feel. If you get off track, do whatever the situation requires to get back to your comfort zone.

ANRED, "Self Help Tips," http://www.anred.com/slf_hlp.html. Used with permission.

Chapter Four

Corne**red**

Cornered

The little girl
looked
for her death in her life,
and her breath couldn't be caught,
and neither
could she,
At least that's what she thought
as she thought
she could eat
and eat
and eat
and not get caught,
but Truth's legs run hard and fast
especially when they belong to God,
and she couldn't
outlast,
outrun them,
She had run
into
her wall,
Cornered,
no matter where she turned,
Truth instead
answered her

by questioning her,
by confronting her,
And she didn't want to answer back,
So
She caught her breath
long enough
to tell her lie,
And deny
that she was
who she was,
Cornered,
And no food
and no lie
could get her out of this one,
She had nowhere else to go,
This little girl's breath
couldn't be caught
and neither could she,
At least
that's what she thought.

At this time, I was obsessed with food, weight, control, and maintaining my secret world. I feared someone discovering my secret obsession—especially the roommates from whom I'd stolen food. I was scared all of the time: scared to be fat, scared to lose control, and scared of being found out. But did that stop me? No. I felt helpless.

I could never eat enough food, but it was always way too much for me to handle. I'd gorge, binge, pig out—whatever you want to call it. The results were still the same: overextended, rock-hard stomach, severe pain and discomfort, and always the sense of failure, shame, and disgust. My heart pounded with panic as I gulped. My hands shook as I stuffed my mouth with enormous quantities of food.

I thought I was hiding my secret well from the outside world. I replenished the food I'd stolen from my roommates. I played "beat the clock" before they came home to notice. I thought they'd never miss what I'd taken. I mean, really, were they going to count every granola bar or measure every cup of rice and cereal? No one does that. Maybe I was safe.

Question: Do you ever steal food or lie concerning food and eating issues?

My roommates, however, *did* notice. It became a regular hide and steal, hide and eat, hide and deny game for me. I tried to be disciplined and reverse the damage, but I had no willpower to control my eating behavior, let alone do what was right. I knew their schedules by heart. I'd wait for them to leave for class. I'd hurry home, skipping my own classes to ensure enough time alone. First, I'd raid stuff that I didn't think was noticeable: a handful of cereal, a three-fingered scoop of peanut butter out of the jar, some cans of soup at the back of the shelf. No one would notice, right? But I couldn't stop. I found myself grabbing anything and taking any amount. I didn't care anymore if they discovered their missing food. I had to eat as much as I could before they came home. When they finally arrived, I fled the apartment or pretended to be asleep, not wanting to deal with the threat of confrontation.

Question: Do you feel you need to hide and isolate yourself from others?

As hard as I tried, I couldn't deny they knew the truth. I felt them look at me and treat me with scorn and accusation. I heard their frustrated sighs. They angrily slammed the refrigerator door and cupboard doors when they discovered their food was missing. Even though I knew their anger was justified, I felt like a monster being hunted, exposed, and trapped! I ignored their reactions, even though they were concerned for me.

Finally, they confronted me. They approached me from time to time saying, "Sheryle, we need to talk." I'd brace myself for each meeting. I was now constantly defensive, feeling that everyone was out to get me. As my roommates questioned me about their missing food, I thought "A-ha! See, that is all you care about. You don't care about me at all." I was beyond seeing the big picture. Anyone reaching out to me was an enemy I needed protection from. I didn't realize that these people were aching to help me but feeling helpless. They didn't know how to deal with my problem any better than I did. To handle the confrontations, I convinced myself I was still in control and played it all off. I'd be cool and deny that there was a problem, while secretly experiencing fear and rage.

Question: Has anyone ever asked you if you are anorexic or bulimic?

I began to receive concerned looks from teachers and class-mates. They gave me looks that said, "I know." One of my guidance counselors asked me to step inside her office as I passed through campus one day. Panic! *She knew.* Scared, I switched into "self-preservation, automatic lying pilot" mode. "Okay, just get through it," I told myself over and over again. Once inside her office, she started out with some initial chit chat, but I felt the ax coming down. This was it: confrontation.

She started to speak, "I'm concerned about you, that you may be bulimic." There! She said it! Even more than fearing my secret obsession would be discovered, I'd feared being labeled as *that* this whole time. Once people found you were anorexic, bulimic, or out of control with food in any way, that would be the only way they would see you. You would stop being a person; you would stop being you. And I didn't want to be thought of that way. I didn't need more reminding of the failure I was at that time. I didn't want people looking at me and judging me only as this "problem," this freakish "disorder." No thanks, no way. Even if I had to lie, I refused to be *that*!

"He who covers his sins will not prosper,
But whoever confesses and forsakes them
will have mercy."
—Proverbs 28:13

So how did I respond to this counselor, who by the way, was a former nun? I lied.

"No, I'm not."

"I'm just concerned about you," she continued carefully.

"I'm fine," still desperately insisting, "I'm okay."

She left it at that.

I left the office feeling triumphant at first, and then it occurred to me: I just lied to a nun. I would now be in deeper trouble with God. But hey, I'd made a life out of lies. I was tangled up in them, why stop now? I'd lied to family, friends, roommates, God—why should a nun be any different? I managed to survive that confrontation, but it made me more guarded, more determined than ever to avoid facing the reality of my disordered life. No, no one would know about this if I could help it!

I couldn't outrun God, though. Even though I felt so removed from Him, He didn't consider Himself removed from me.

A **Prayer** to Rise
For the One Who Needs to Approach a Loved One

Father, I come to You in the name of Jesus, asking for help in my life. Thank You, Lord, that You are a God of miraculous compassion and wisdom. I ask You to empower me with these blessings now as I lift up my loved one (insert loved one's name here).

Lord, You know the pain and concern I feel when I look at her. I am scared for her life and well-being, and I am at a loss about what to do next in the face of this disorder. I ask You to help me. Give me the compassionate, loving words of wisdom to speak when I approach her.

I pray for help, for support, and for encouragement from others as we pursue Your divine health and freedom. Inspire open communication and unconditional love and support for everyone concerned in this matter. Touch our lives in real ways so we can all heal. I ask this in Jesus's name. Amen.

Journaling Section

To Help You **Work Through** Your Thoughts

For the One Who Needs to Approach a Loved One

Has your loved one displayed signs of disordered behavior regarding food, weight, body issues, and dieting?

_____

_____

Has your loved one ever lied to you concerning such issues?

_____

_____

_____

_____

Has she isolated herself socially and/or from family functions? List several examples.

_____

_____

_____

_____

Do eating disorders (anorexia, bulimia, compulsive overeating) run in her family? In your family?

_____

_____

_____

Do you yourself have issues regarding food or weight? How do you address them around your loved one?

_____

_____

_____

_____

_____

How is the spiritual health of her family? How would you rate your own spiritual health?

_____

_____

_____

_____

_____

_____

Do you blame her, yourself, God, or anyone else for what is happening? Do you see it as sin? A sickness? What are your feelings regarding your loved one?

_____

_____

_____

Are you connected with a church body? A youth center specializing in eating disorders? What pastors or counselors are available to you?

_____

_____

_____

_____

Does your family have issues with keeping secrets? Are you willing to engage in open communication and truthful discussion? Are you willing to pursue Christian therapy?

_____

_____

_____

Scripture to Consider

Proverbs 28:13

When You Want to Help Someone You Care About

What to Do...

If your child is younger than 18

- Get professional help immediately. You have a legal and moral responsibility to get your child the care she or he needs. Don't let tears, tantrums, or promises to do better stop you. Begin with a physical exam and psychological evaluation.
- If the physician recommends hospitalization, do it. People die from these disorders, and sometimes they need a structured time-out to break entrenched patterns.
- If the counselor asks you to participate in family sessions, do so. Children spend only a few hours a week with their counselors. The rest of the time they live with their families. You need as many tools as you can get to help your child learn new ways of coping with life.

If your friend is younger than 18

- Tell a trusted adult—parent, teacher, coach, pastor, school nurse, school counselor, etc.—about your concern. If you don't, you may unwittingly help your friend avoid the treatment she or he needs to get better.
- Even though it would be hard, consider telling your friend's parents why you are concerned. That friend might be hiding unhealthy behaviors from them, and they deserve to know so they can arrange help and treatment. If you cannot bear to do this yourself, ask your parents or perhaps the school nurse for help.

Continued on next page.

If the person is older than 18

- Legally the person is now an adult and can refuse treatment if not ready to change. Nevertheless, reach out.
- Tell her or him that you are concerned. Be gentle.
- Suggest that there has to be a better way to deal with life than starving and stuffing.
- Encourage person to use professional help, but expect resistance and denial. You can lead a horse to water, but...

Things to Do

- Talk to the person when you are calm, not frustrated or emotional. Be kind. The person is probably ashamed and fears criticism and rejection.
- Mention evidence you have heard or seen that suggests disordered eating, without dwelling on appearance or weight. Instead talk about health, relationships (withdrawal?), and mood.
- Realize the person will not change until she wants to.
- Provide information. ANRED is one good source (http://www.anred.com).
- Be supportive and caring. Be a good listener and give advice only when asked. Even then, be prepared to have it ignored.
- Continue to suggest professional help. Don't pester, but don't give up.
- Ask, "Is what you are doing really working to get you what you want?"
- Talk about the advantages of recovery and a normal life.

- Agree that recovery is hard, but emphasize that many people have recovered.
- If the person is too frightened to see a counselor, offer to go with her or him the first time.
- Realize that recovery is the person's responsibility, not yours.
- Resist guilt. Do the best you can and then be gentle with yourself.

Things Not to Do
- Never nag, plead, beg, bribe, threaten, or manipulate. These things don't work.
- Avoid power struggles. You will lose.
- Never criticize or shame. These tactics are cruel, and the person will withdraw.
- Don't pry. Respect privacy.
- Don't be a food monitor. You will create resentment and distance in the relationship.
- Don't try to control. The person will withdraw and ultimately outwit you.
- Don't waste time trying to reassure your friend that she is not fat. Your friend will not be convinced.
- Don't get involved in endless conversations about weight, food, and calories. They make matters worse.
- Don't give advice unless asked.
- Don't expect the person to follow your advice even if she asked for it.
- Don't say, "You are too thin." She will secretly celebrate.

Continued on next page.

- Don't say, "It's good you have gained weight." She will lose it.
- Don't let the person always decide when, what, and where you will eat. She should not control everything, every time.
- Don't ignore stolen food and evidence of purging. Insist on responsibility.
- Don't overestimate what you can accomplish.

Adapted from ANRED, "When You Want to Help Someone You Care About," http://www.anred.com/hlp.html. Used with permission.

Chapter Five

The Merry-**Go-Round**

The "Around We Go" Merry-Go-Round

Another trip, another ride
on the "around we go" merry-go-round,
The answer solution salvation
stopped being
the answer solution salvation
long ago,
Insanity charges admission
with promises disguised
as hope
future
life,
But they never are
they never were,
None of these could ever be God
Another trip, another ride
on the "around we go" merry-go-round,
Moving in circles
doesn't get her anywhere
except
dizzy
confused,
And all she wanted to do
was stop,
Not necessarily

matters
of life and death,
Rather
Matters
of life and nonlife,
And she definitely
wasn't
living
or being
She was instead
Eating
Dieting
Riding
Another trip
Another ride
The "around we go" merry-go-round
stopped being
The answer solution salvation
long ago
It never was,
And so
She let God stop the ride.

After my confrontation with the counselor, my life took a dangerous turn. My binge eating habits began to show physically. The many "just one time" gorge sessions were becoming obvious. In the next few weeks, 80 pounds became 100 pounds (the unacceptable three-digit weight). As the number kept climbing, I couldn't stop eating.

I became desperate to do whatever it took to stop my increasing weight. I couldn't use the vomiting form of purging. To me, vomiting represented being sick, and being sick was an unacceptable option. The incident with my dad, at age 14, taught me that being sick represented weakness, laziness, and worthlessness. I *wasn't* sick. I was just doing damage control. I abused water pills (without water), laxatives, and hours of grueling exercise after each one of my binges. Punishment was the key word for me here. I had to make myself pay!

Question: Do you feel the need to punish yourself?

Even though I was putting my body through the trauma of repeated bingeing, purging, and rapid weight gain, my mental state was more dangerous. I crossed from just shame, disgust, and guilt into believing I was unforgivable and hopeless. Previously I welcomed death, believing that I would be with God enjoying the peace and rest I'd been wanting for so long. But now I believed that if I died, I would deserve only hell. And I would be in torment forever.

As I ate myself to death, I accepted this inevitable hell. I believed that I was damned, doomed, cursed from the start. I was too much of a failure for even God, who now seemed to be as far away as possible. He wasn't answering my prayers, tears, or cries. I began yelling to myself: "Why should He?" I was beyond saving grace.

In my hopeless desperation, I even consulted a psychic hot-line. I was desperate for any good news for my predicament. It was just another attempt at a God substitute. The call only made matters worse, and not just because of the phone bill. I felt that I had crossed over a line somewhere. I knew it was wrong, but I was desperate for any hope anyone could give me. I didn't find hope there either.

Question: Do you find yourself looking to other sources to alleviate pain and promote happiness for yourself?

Desperate for any comfort now, I'd repeatedly eat "one last feast," trying to give myself the satisfaction that I'd eaten absolutely everything I could possibly desire. Then I'd be "full enough," and I'd never have to do this again. My "last feasts" led to erratic, desperate behaviors.

Question: Do you make promises to yourself and to others that you cannot keep?

In a desperate attempt to recapture control after each "last time," I did something that would confuse and anger anyone in a third world country: I threw away all of the food. Suddenly, taking out the trash became my favorite chore. I'd gather and dispose of anything and everything that could tempt me, and I'd dump it in the trash. I couldn't have it, any of it, around me. This included my roommates' food as well. The refrigerator and cupboard doors slammed even louder now, as my roommates' frustration levels increased. Nothing they did or said seemed to make things better. I knew they would confront me, but my desperate compulsion to "get rid of the food" took over. Hurry! Hurry! Before it's too late. Get rid of it now! I'd be first to volunteer among my roommates to take out the trash, because I knew what "goodies" I'd thrown out. Only after tossing all of the food into the huge dumpster could I feel victory, freedom, and relief. It was over. I could go back inside and temporarily feel good, even satisfied and safe for a while.

Question: Do you prefer to eat alone?

Inevitably though, after a few hours or a few days, my cravings would begin. Of course, there was no food anywhere inside my apartment. In the trash dumpster, though, sat many wonderful goodies! Yes, that's it. I'd simply get the stuff I'd thrown away. I knew that I could find everything I'd thrown out.

Trips to the dumpster at 2:30 A.M. were not unusual. I'd usually make up some excuse to go out (I need to check the mail at 11:45 P.M.). I rummaged through the dumpster. Where was that ice cream I threw out? Where were those cookies? I'd dig through the bag, eating whatever "leftovers" I could on the spot. If I couldn't find my stuff, I'd rummage through other people's trash bags. You'd be amazed at what "perfectly good food" people would throw away. Of course, it may have been "perfectly good" at the time it was thrown out. Now, it was garbage. When you're sick and hungry though, semantics don't mean much. I'm still amazed I never experienced food poisoning during these times. I lost count of all of the times I ate runny melted ice cream or frozen yogurt that had been in the dump for days. Luckily, the frigid Minnesota weather refrigerated much of the trash I ate.

I was caught on more than one occasion. I'd try to play it off, pretending everything was normal as people passed by me scrounging in the dumpster. As I became more desperate, however, I began going to the dumpster frequently in broad daylight while other students were coming and going from class. I was in full-blown denial as I tried to convince myself I could "just act natural" and disguise the truth. I tried to act like I was rearranging the garbage in the dumpster to make room for the trash I'd just taken out. You know those pesky dumpsters. They're always so full. Sometimes I tried the "oops, I dropped something in the garbage, and I must fish it out" excuse. I had dropped something all right: my guard, my dignity. How could any excuse explain me chowing down on dinner à la Hefty bag? How would eating a mouthful of tossed-out cookies and crackers help me in my search for my "lost" apartment keys? Sick. But I wasn't sick—oh, no! I was just getting some fresh air.

I felt so much shame. Shame was one thing when I was by myself. But when someone else's eyes were watching me, knowing that what I was doing was sick, it was totally different. I was sinking—daily, being pulled further into hell. This was my life now: gluttony, sickness, desperation, fear, hurt, self-hatred, chaos, defeat, and discovery. Not exactly the "damage control" I was after. I couldn't hide any longer from others what I was doing, who I was becoming. It was obvious, and people were noticing.

September passed into October, and I continued to gain weight. At first, I could conceal it. I was still enough underweight that my baggy clothes were still baggy on me. They concealed my enlarged stomach, and I felt safe and protected in my armor. But soon, my disguising layers stopped working for me. I was in despair as with each passing day, the big sweatshirts and baggy jeans became tighter and tighter. Soon, nothing I owned fit. Believe me, there's only so much you can do with sweats. My desperation and increasingly limited wardrobe made my self-image worse.

I ate with more fury, recklessness, hopelessness—and denial. I quickly passed through the forbidden 100-pound mark all the

way to a noticeable 140 pounds by mid-October. I'd
pounds in a month and a half. I was devastated, hor
defeated. Still, I couldn't stop. I kept gaining.

Quickly, I climbed to 150, 160, 170, 180 pounds. The weight
showed up first on my stomach. It wasn't necessarily weight so
much as it was an overextended stomach from binge after binge.
The weight showed up next in my legs. After reading a few books
on eating disorders out of curiosity, I learned this was a normal
starting point. You need to have a firm base to stand on. Initially,
the muscle that I had starved off my body was being replaced.
As I kept bingeing on high-fat food, however, I found myself
with the fat legs I once had. They felt different now, though.
Physically, it felt as if my leg veins and my very skin itself were
being stretched tight and on the verge of ripping apart.

The weight showed up next on my face. Puffy "chipmunk"
cheeks replaced the hollow, defined cheekbones I'd worked for.
Puffiness in general replaced my gaunt, sharp facial features. I'd
lost my sharp jawline and had acquired a double chin. Each
morning I woke up and starred in horror at this fat girl's face.
My hips, my arms, all my parts were now dramatically different.
I'd had months of seeing myself thin, but now I was heavier
than I had ever been in my life.

By May, I reached 190 pounds. I stopped weighing myself. In
less than a year, I had undergone a 100-pound weight gain.
People still expressed concern, but it was now because of my
obesity. This was what I was trying to avoid in the first place,
being the fat girl.

Question: Do you experience rapid weight fluctuations?

I was determined. I'd lost weight before, and I'd do it again. I was
transferring to a new school, and I wanted to reinvent myself.

So that summer I began a new attempt at dieting. I was racing against time here. I had three months to trade in my hideous 190-pound frame for something more acceptable. I reverted back to my old ways as much as I could. However, my body had gotten used to eating again. Imagine that. Human beings, by God's design, have to put up with some pesky little habits—and eating is one of them.

I made sure that I was away from my parents and their home all summer. I wanted no interference with my plans. I didn't need a hovering mother and critical father threatening my goals. I hadn't returned home to them since that previous summer when I weighed 80 pounds. Returning home this heavy now meant that I'd lost and they'd won. My pride and ego wouldn't admit defeat.

Question: Do you weigh yourself often (at least once a day or several times a day)?

Three months lay before me. My usual approach of exercising more while eating less was once again the name of the game. I kept the calorie list each day. Was I a good girl? Was I a bad girl? I could only keep up the calorie counting and exercise for so many days. Then those tempting foods would start calling my name again. Regardless of what I was telling myself, I was feeling desperate for comfort food. And so I ate. It went beyond a cookie, a cracker, or a chip. I devoured bags of them in one sitting. As I ravenously ate, I thought, *Just this once. I'll get back on track tomorrow.* I lived this way for a month and a half. Summer was ticking away. More pressure came with each passing day and each passing feast.

By mid-July, I was far from my ideal. I'd managed to lose some weight; I was about 175 pounds now. It wasn't good enough, though. As I looked to September, I'd get scared and yet more determined. This was my big chance to be a new, acceptable me. I couldn't afford to blow it. I didn't want anyone in my new life to know anything about who I'd been. I didn't want to be seen or known as the fat girl, the anorexic, or the bulimic. I just wanted to be seen and known as Sheryle.

So I began my desperate, last-ditch effort to lose weight. I decided after one comfort-food session to eat nothing until either I'd lost what I'd wanted or arrived at my new school. That was it, no food. And so, from the middle of July to early September, I consumed only cans of diet soda and a cough drop now and then. I spent my grocery money on 12- or 24-pack cases of diet soda or water. Once again, I was tired. I'd think about Jesus during His 40-day wilderness fast. Believe me, I wanted to turn my diet soda into bread so many times. But my goals, my pride, my "new life" wouldn't let me. So, irritable and tired, I slept as much as I could.

Question: Do you ever stop eating completely for periods of time?

When September did come, I was at 150 pounds, and more than ready to get to school. Whether I was physically able or not was debatable. Moving my stuff out of my summer apartment and into my new, third-floor dorm room was more than I could physically do. Up and down with trunks, suitcases, and boxes—I was winded from the start. Mom "caught" me on this. She had remarked on more than one occasion about my weight loss with a critical, "Oh no, here we go again." Before she left on moving day, she confronted and reprimanded me with her usual, "You better eat something." I responded to her with my usual lies, "I will, I am eating, I'm fine."

With her gone, I felt relief. I was here. I was in my new beginning, my new life, my new self. In the back of my mind, I still had the screaming thought, *Don't bet on it, fat girl. You better not blow it this time!* Pressure.

When I did resume eating, I was so careful, eating diet foods and drinking diet sodas constantly. I reached 140, then 130 pounds. I seemed to level off there. I never did get down to my "ideal" 80- or even 90-pound goal. My metabolism was shot; my body wasn't doing it anymore. I was stuck. I limited myself to diet soda (preferably with caffeine in it for energy and for its diuretic effect) and LifeSavers candy (ironic, huh?). I'd do this as long as I could until my next failure. I tried harder as I continued to spin on an endless merry-go-round of wacky diets. On my "candy-only" diet I could live on suckers, spice drops, and Hot Tamale candy for a month.

Question: Do you eliminate certain foods or eat only certain foods as part of a diet plan?

When I turned 21, I tried an "alcohol" diet. I decided that I could be full, entertained, and social by drinking. Drinking on an empty stomach, however, made my tolerance level dangerously low. With one Bloody Mary or Margarita, I was impaired and would fall into giggling fits. This "diet" didn't last long. As a high-calorie depressant, it was lowering my metabolism and making me fatter, bloated, and puffy. In addition to affecting my appearance, I had a scary blackout session one New Year's Eve. After waking up fully dressed in a bathtub, I could not remember anything that happened the previous night. This was quite a deterrent to someone who prized control.

Even though I saw the danger of my alcohol diet, I was blind to the other deadly decisions I was making. I began seriously contemplating using an addictive substance as a diet aid. All sorts of "solutions" popped up. Diet pills and caffeine tablets gave me both an energy charge and the illusion of weight loss, due to their diuretic effects. Thankfully I never tried smoking, although I knew it was a common method of dieting. I had family members and friends who became hooked on cigarettes while trying to lose weight. It suppressed their appetites and gave them "something to do with their hands." It also gave one of them cancer. She passed away a few years ago from it.

Question: Do you ever engage in other behaviors (smoking, drinking alcohol, drugs) to cope in your life?

All my diets produced the same yo-yo results. I'd lose weight and feel deprived, grouchy, hungry. I'd then eat for comfort and release and, therefore, gain weight once again. I constantly lost and gained the same 15 to 20 pounds, weighing anywhere from 135 to 155 pounds. Although my weight fluctuations weren't as severe as they'd been when I was 19 and 20 years old, the process was still desperate and depressing. I never felt satisfied where I was, and I certainly never felt I was at my "right weight."

I was on a spiritual merry-go-round as well. Did God hate me? Did He think of me as a hopeless failure? I began to wonder whether I was saved or damned. Did I lose my soul somewhere because of these eating disorders? Had I gone too far?

Seeing myself as His daughter seemed impossible. I couldn't do that with my father, how was I going to even start with an omnipotent Creator? But now, in the midst of all of this disorder, anger, guilt, shame, ugliness, and desperation, I found myself tired and wanting Him more than anything I'd ever wanted before. I wanted God to be real for me, but I felt that the eating disorders stood in my way. To say that I was confused and filled with doubt would be an understatement. I felt constantly surrounded by evil that was seeking to destroy me. Weird stuff, I know. And all this from dieting, you may ask?

For most people, the issue of dieting is a simple, harmless one. But for some people, it is a dangerous risk. It's like Russian roulette. You can choose to play the game, but you can't guarantee how it will turn out for you. I had no idea that the innocent diet I initially started would bring me to such agonizing, paralyzing lows. I had no idea that when I started this whole diet merry-go-round, I would find myself at the mercy of these evil lies.

Be careful. Be careful what you allow yourself to believe. Know this: Your answer is not in any strategy, plan, or eating disorder. Your answer is in God.

For You have formed my inward parts;
You have covered me in my mother's womb."
—*Psalm 139:13*

Question: Are you always on a diet?

I had to make a decision. The merry-go-round and the endless yo-yoing were too much. I made a decision that gradually impacted everything in my world. I decided, *Fine God, if others know about this, fine. I'm tired.* I now felt deeply excavated, lying dormant and waiting for death. As I was lying in bed, the picture of Jesus with Jairus's daughter flashed back to me. Like her, I was dead to so many things. I remembered all the times my thin self, my overweight self, and my every-in-between-stage self felt like nothing more than a hopeless, dead girl. I was tired on so many levels and dismissed it, at first, as just being exhaustion on my part.

And then, I remembered…"Little girl, I say to you, arise."

"'Little girl, I say to you, arise.'"
—Mark 5:41

A **Prayer** to Rise

Father, I come to You in the name of Jesus, asking for help in my life. Thank You, Lord, that You are my answer, no matter what the problem or situation may be. I pray that You will be this to me now.

Lord, You know that I've tried every diet, every approach, some even that are dangerous and extreme. I've tried everything I know in pursuit of my goal to be a certain weight and size. Forgive me, Lord, for looking to and placing power and glory toward these diets and methods. I confess that I've resorted to unhealthy, dangerous extremes that have not glorified and pleased You. Forgive me for not taking better care of the temple You've given me. Empower me, by Your grace, to change not only my behaviors, but my desires as well.

"Let the words of my mouth and the meditation of my heart be acceptable in Your sight, O LORD, my strength and my redeemer" (Psalm 19:14).

Lord, help me to stop this unfruitful way of living and help me live my life the way You desire me to live it for You. In Jesus's name, I pray. Amen.

Journaling Section

To Help You **Work Through** Your Thoughts

Do you feel you deserve to be happy? If not, why not? Do you believe God wants you to be happy? If your answer is "no," why not?

_____

_____

_____

_____

_____

What are your weight fluctuations like?

_____

_____

_____

_____

How often do you weigh yourself?

_____

What are your feelings before you weigh yourself? After you weigh yourself?

_____

_____

_____

_____

How do you feel when you lose weight? Gain weight?

_____

_____

_____

_____

What is the longest period of time you've gone without eating? How did you feel during this time?

_____

_____

What foods have you eliminated completely from your diet? What are your "rules" concerning certain foods?

_____

_____

_____

_____

Do you participate in other habits (drinking alcohol, smoking cigarettes, doing drugs, shopping) to cope in your life? How do they compare with eating and/or dieting?

_____

_____

_____

_____

_____

List below all of the diets you've been on in your life. State when you were on them, what results (positive or negative) occurred, and how you felt while on the diet.

Type of Diet	Duration	Result	How I Felt

Scripture to Consider

Psalm 139:13

Signs That You May Be a Compulsive Eater/ Dieter
(Author's Personal Experience)

- You repeatedly go on crash diets.
- Your weight fluctuates constantly.
- Your sense of success or failure is determined mainly by weight loss.
- You are critical of yourself, your body, or your physical appearance.
- You speak negatively about yourself.
- You are secretive about your behavior.
- You are ashamed of your behavior.
- You are convinced that there is something wrong with you and your struggle with weight.
- You isolate yourself from family, friends, and social gatherings.
- You struggle with depression and anger.

Chapter Six

Fears
(The Worst Did **Not** Happen)

Worst Case Scenario (This One Meal)

She sat down and ate,
not everything in the world
but something,
No bigger than the size of her dinner plate,
She sat down and ate
one meal,
and this one meal
suddenly
didn't make her fat.
The worst case scenario
didn't happen.
This one meal
didn't make her world end,
She was still here,
She was still
under God's grace,
Maybe
it was just
fear.
Maybe
It was just
food,

no more power
than that.
Maybe
she was okay,
Worst case scenario
didn't happen,
She
was still
intact,
far
far
far
from hell,
She ate
this one meal,
She was okay
God loved her
after all,
Worst case scenario
It didn't happen
It didn't happen.

"'Little girl, I say to you, arise.'"
—Jesus, in Mark 5:41

As I was wishing that Jesus had said that to me, a new thought occurred. How do I know that He didn't? This new thought threw me! Why would He say this to me? I had done and been so many horrible things. As far as I was concerned, I was on my way to hell. But I couldn't shake the thoughts of this story. Was there hope that I wasn't doomed after all?

I became intrigued with the story of Jairus's daughter. The images from the miniseries of Jesus's life constantly played in my mind. Every time I lay down to sleep, I'd think about the story. It wouldn't leave me alone. My soul was in a tug of war. For so long, I'd just accepted believing I was bound for hell. Now, all of a sudden, that familiar thought had competition. Maybe hope was possible for me again.

I'd never really been much of a Bible reader. I'd look at the thick book and think, "That's too much reading. It's too difficult—too many thous and thines—and besides, it doesn't really apply to me." But now, it applied to me.

Of course, I had no clue where to find the story. I had to do some hunting. I narrowed it down to the New Testament. Hey, that's where the stories about Jesus are found, right? Sooner or later, I'd have to come across this little girl.

As I plowed through the Bible, I found a Scripture that summed up who I was and what I was going through.

"'Lord, I believe; help my unbelief!'"
—Mark 9:24

That was me! I knew I couldn't be enough, love enough, believe enough, and have faith enough unless God *helped* me.

When I began to feel that I wasn't hell-bound after all, I experienced an opposing tug in this battle. Another thought popped up: *How do you know you even believe in God…or want to believe in God?* This scared me. My life showed me repeatedly that I couldn't trust my own heart. Maybe this desperation for God was a new lie.

I decided to fight as hard as I could, not because I was nobly seeking after God, but because I was scared to death of my life without Him. I had to find this story of Jairus's daughter, but more than that, I had to find God Himself.

The guilt and shame over my past took a backseat to my new urgency in finding God. Some days, I felt like I was saved and on my way to a wonderful life with God. Other days, I left the lights on and slept clutching my Bible for dear life, like a child clutches a teddy bear. I cried. I laughed. I shouted. I cowered. I whispered and whimpered. But through it all, I kept praying, "God, be real to me, be real." And I kept reading the Bible.

I finally found the story in **Mark 5:21–24, 35–43**. It started out with desperate parents wanting their daughter healed. I could relate. My own family wanted me cured, fixed. In the Bible story, Jairus, a ruler of the synagogue, begged Jesus to come and heal his daughter, who was at the point of death. Jesus agreed to go with him. But before Jesus could get there, some people came from Jairus's house and told Jairus not to bring Jesus; there was no longer any point.

"'Your daughter is dead.
Why trouble the Teacher any further?'"
—Mark 5:35

I could relate. There were so many people who had given up on me. I heard their voices and frustrated sighs: "It's hopeless, she'll never change." But then, as I continued reading, it jumped out at me:

"As soon as Jesus heard the word that was spoken, He said to the ruler of the synagogue, 'Do not be afraid; only believe.'"
—Mark 5:36

He *ignored* their comments? He didn't listen to them? Hope started in me as I continued to read. He wouldn't let anyone else come along with Him, to argue with Him. I looked at my life. For so long, my life was about seeking a substitute for God, instead of seeking God Himself. I'd turned to food, accomplishment, image, people, and things. But it was Jesus this whole time. Jesus was my answer, my answer to pain, to fear, to Father.

"'I am the way, the truth, and the life. No one comes to the Father except through Me.'"
—Jesus, in John 14:6

Jesus entered the house where people were weeping and wailing. He said to them, "The child is not dead, but sleeping" (Mark 5:39). I thought about how death had become my life.

I'd focused on death as the beauty, the answer. Stuffing and starving myself was death. Bingeing, purging, punishing—all were death. But what if these words could apply to me and the death I was going through? What if anorexia, bulimia, compulsive eating—what if none of them were the final word? What if Jesus was? What if the Bible really was true?

I read on through **Mark 5:41**: "**Then He took the child by the hand, and said to her, 'Talitha, cumi,' which is translated, 'Little girl, I say to you, arise.'**"

And she did! What if I could arise from all of this, too? What if I could wake up and live beyond anorexia, bulimia, overeating, and food and weight concerns? And then, to top it all off, I read at the end of the story in **Mark 5:43**, Jesus "**said that something should be given her to eat.**"

I felt that I was that little girl. You mean Jesus wants me to eat? Not starve, not stuff myself either, but eat something? I didn't have to starve or binge? "Something"—everything in moderation? You mean Jesus said it first?

That's how two new journeys began for me: adapting my approach to eating and adapting my approach to life and truth. Neither was a neat little process of starting and finishing step one, step two, etc. I discovered just how patient, gradual, and merciful God can be. I faced the fears of my worst case scenario on two fronts: 1) the fear of food, eating, and my views toward exercise, and 2) the fear of letting people know my secrets. It's difficult to say which scared me more. However, I knew if I wanted my relationship with God to be real, I needed to do this.

I changed my eating habits over time. In fact, I'm still changing them (a part of the process). I began to look at food for what it was: a gift from God designed to keep His creation alive. Food was not designed to be entertainment, comfort, or a God substitute. He did mean for food to be enjoyable—hey, taste buds, right?

I faced a new question: How do I enjoy food as simply food and nothing else? Through prayer, fasting, and curiosity, God led me to information—tidbits and books—on nutrition and on what food does for the physical body (what it was meant to do). I faced my fear of food—my belief that it would automatically make me fat. It wasn't an all-or-nothing deal. Food had no more power than what I'd chosen to give it.

Question: Are you afraid of food? Have you chosen to give food too much power in your life?

Although I was seeking out practical, livable answers on my own, I needed outside help. My first help came through a naturopathic doctor. I sought her out shortly after I moved from Minnesota to Oregon. I wasn't feeling well after I moved, and I was concerned. With help from the doctor, I found out I needed to make several changes. I had already gotten rid of a few bad habits, like drinking sodas. I ate chemical-free food as much as I could, avoiding sugar and preservatives. Although I felt better, I still felt "run down."

The doctor had me chart what I was eating daily. My eyes were opened to how I was eating. I would eat only one large meal a day and then feel overstuffed and lethargic. The doctor explained why. All of my energy focused on digesting this meal, which was usually larger than my fist-sized stomach. This was not what God had intended at all. Ideally, food should boost your energy level, not drain it. I found that smaller meals dispersed frequently throughout the day made me feel energized, satisfied, and in better spirits, even hopeful.

The most valuable lesson I learned was how to listen to my own body. What did hungry feel like? Not starving or ravenous, as I'd previously been, but rather what did being physically hungry feel like? What did satisfied feel like? Not stuffed, not overfed, but satisfied. This was all new to me. Over time, I ate in such a way that was not only making me feel better but look better as well. Since I wasn't starving, I didn't have the desire to binge. Since I wasn't bingeing, I could enjoy feeling normal afterward. I wasn't uncomfortable, in pain or drained. And I didn't have the bloated, distended stomach either. I didn't look like I was nine months pregnant. I just looked like me. Yes, I actually felt good! I now was having energy—and the desire—to live.

In time, I started becoming more relaxed around food. This was big for me. My digestive system wasn't tied up in anxious knots over what I was eating. No longer did I have to gulp food and race against some restrictive time frame. I found myself eating until I was satisfied—even if that meant that there were leftovers. Yes, leftovers! Not having to eat everything on my plate right then and there was a new concept for me. I could come back to it later if I chose, another new concept. For so long, my "never again" approach to eating was my "answer" for avoiding being fat. However, this wasn't the case at all. I would eat again and be okay the next day. Eating meals didn't automatically make me fat overnight. I looked the same. I know that this is a no-brainer to most people, but it really turned a light on for me. I could eat and not be fat. I could eat and be okay.

Question: Do you believe food—any food at all—will make you fat?

My attitude toward exercise began relaxing too. I had previously had an "or else" view of exercise, full of "musts" and oppressive rules. My exercise routine had been measured by strict quotas of thousands of sit-ups and hours of "punishment." To me, exercise was a jail sentence for my crime of eating "too much," eating in general, and just being myself. I was afraid of the consequences I'd have to face if I didn't do my routine punishment exactly or perfectly.

Question: Do you pressure yourself to exercise, or do you actually enjoy it?

My desire for the six-hour-a-day routine was gone. I was burned out on it. So I went from exercising six grueling hours every day to just one to two hours. Occasionally, I'd even miss a day. *And the next day, I was still okay!* I found out that it was actually healthy to skip exercise at least one day a week. Physiologically, the human body needs at least one day of rest a week in order to repair the damage of living an active life. I then "took off" Sundays—God's Sabbath. This was encouraging, and soon I took the entire weekend off. I also took off holidays. Gone were the Christmases and Thanksgivings and Easters spent working out. I actually enjoyed the holiday without guilt and without my "must exercise" attitude. I felt freer than I had in a long time.

"'I have come that they may have life,
and that they may have it more abundantly.'"
—Jesus, in John 10:10

Jesus gives life and life more abundantly. No, it didn't say in the Bible, exercise more abundantly, do sit-ups more abundantly, arm curls, push-ups, laps around the track more abundantly, it says *life* more abundantly. To quote the T-shirt and bumper sticker, I had to "get a life."

I started accepting myself—and not just in terms of my physical being. God was letting me discover that I didn't have to be anxious all of the time. In fact, God didn't want me to be anxious any of the time. Little by little, I started becoming less afraid. I was shocked because I thought that it would be this dramatic transformation. I was waiting to be "perfectly finished" already. I learned that, as a card-carrying member of the human race, there is no such thing. I learned that I'm still a work in progress, and that's okay. God, I guess, was and is working on me bit by bit, eating disorders and all.

> "'For My thoughts are not your thoughts,
> Nor are your ways My ways,' says the LORD.
> 'For as the heavens are higher than the earth,
> So are My ways higher than your ways,
> And My thoughts than your thoughts.'"
> —Isaiah 55:8–9

I thought, initially, I could do it all, including my relationship with God, all by myself. That thought, too, was wrong! As I continued praying and reading the Bible, I found myself wanting more than just this limited life. I desperately wanted to be

in a church now. That took me by surprise. I'd had no real experience growing up feeling connected to anyone, let alone,
a church, with people and everything! This is when God really
started interrupting my life, as He did some rearranging.

Question: Is your life filled with loving family, friends, and
activities that interest you?

As my diet and exercise routines were stabilizing more, as my
health was improving under the care of my doctor, I found
myself becoming more comfortable with the next step in this
whole process: disclosure. Again, as it seems to be the case with
me, God was dealing very slowly, very gradually with me. It was
during this slow gradual process I began not only to learn but
to live the wonderful reality of **John 8:32: "The truth shall
make you free."**

> "'If you abide in My word, . . .
> you shall know the truth,
> and the truth shall make you free.'"
> —Jesus, in John 8:31–32

Of all of the things I've thought I would be, I never thought free
would be one of them. I guess when it comes to God, never say
never.

A **Prayer** to Rise

Father, I come to You in the name of Jesus, asking for help in my life. Thank You, Lord, that You are a God of love and power, greater than any fear I could ever experience.

Lord, You know all of the fears I'm dealing with right now. I feel paralyzed and overwhelmed by them. I've made wrong choices in response to them. I ask for forgiveness now in Jesus's name. Help me to not be afraid, for You haven't given me **"a spirit of fear, but of power and of love and of a sound mind"** (2 Timothy 1:7). Help me to live Your promising victory.

Lord, give me courage to face and forgive others and myself for situations and events that I can't change. Free me from the fear of rejection and of being hurt, comforting me always with Your love and divine presence.

I thank You that You are empowering me to live beyond my limiting fears to Your limitless love. I receive it now by faith, in Jesus's name. Amen.

Journaling Section

To Help You **Work Through** Your Thoughts

Do you feel unacceptable, even to God, right now? If so why?

_____

_____

_____

_____

_____

_____

_____

Do you see God as a loving God? Why or why not?

_____

_____

_____

_____

_____

_____

_____

Do you believe any food will make you fat?

_____

_____

_____

_____

_____

_____

_____

_____

What happens if you don't exercise? How do you feel?

_____

_____

_____

_____

_____

_____

_____

_____

How do you feel about your place with family and friends? What role do you play when you're around them (the good girl, the athlete, the brain)?

_____

_____

_____

_____

_____

_____

What are you most afraid of? What do you think God can do concerning your fears?

_____

_____

_____

_____

_____

_____

Scriptures to Consider

Mark 9:24   John 8:32
Mark 5:35–43   John 14:6
Isaiah 55:8–9   2 Timothy 1:7

Tips for Overcoming Your Fears
(Author's Personal Experience)

- Recognize nothing is as bad as it seems. There is no "end-all, be-all"—or else—to life. Life is a process.
- Realize that everyone deals with fear. Don't beat yourself up for being afraid. Remember: Courage is doing something you are afraid to do.
- Try new things, even things that scare you.
- Don't worry about failing. You will fail at some things. You will make mistakes. That doesn't make you a failure.
- Start taking small steps, small risks. The important thing is to start!
- Be open to knowing and to being known, to learning about others and having people learn about you. You are incredible and worth discovering!
- Be patient with yourself. Remember, it's all a process.
- Forgive yourself and others. Fear and unforgiveness often go together, keeping you imprisoned. Give grace to others who have their own struggles and issues.
- Pray. Prayer works. Pray for help, for wisdom, for courage to face your fears.
- Receive the love God wants to give you. No matter what, you are worthy of love.

Chapter Seven

Disclosure
(The Cat Is Out of the Bag)

The Cat Is Out of the Bag

A terrified animal
trapped by cornered corners
of my own making,
I wasn't taking
any chances,
any risks,
as I'd lie to myself, God, and anyone
who came near me,
I feared vulnerability,
I was afraid to let
anyone
see
me,
But now
I wanted to be
more than this animal,
more
than this terror.
I had to let go
of the terrified
trapped

cornered animal
with all of her corner secrets
she'd trapped herself into,
I had to let
the cat out of the bag
in order to begin
to be free.
I had to let go
of licking my wounds
long enough
to let God begin healing
me,
I had to let go
of the hiding
long enough
in order to see
that God's love
was all
around and for
me,
And yes,
telling
the truth
to myself,
to God,
to anyone
was truly
beginning
and continuing
to set me free.
The cat was out of the bag,
clawing and scratching

no longer,
I now had hands of prayer
as God showed me
His love was always there,
A terrified
trapped
cornered animal no longer,
I was finally me,
And God knew it
all along.

> *"'For I will restore health to you*
> *And heal you of your wounds,' says the LORD."*
> *—Jeremiah 30:17*

Disclosure was the next step in my recovery process. As I was focusing on the benefits of physical health again, I desired to address my emotional and spiritual needs as well. Again, this pursuit was not tied up in a neat package. Disclosure would be experimental for me, "trying it out" on people, testing the waters.

Question: Are you scared for people to know "the real you"?

My first successful attempt at disclosure occurred at a doctor's visit. I thought, *She's a doctor; I'm her patient. She needs to know these things.* Although it was a small step, I felt relieved and empowered as I filled out the medical history forms. I was still nervous, though, as I wrote that I was recovering from eating disorders in the "Other Conditions" blank.

When we were in the exam room, going over my history, I felt relief when she barely batted an eyelash at my "horrible secrets." I don't know what I feared. Would she gasp in horror, alert her staff and the local media, sequester me to a cell for the rest of my life, while telling me how worthless, hopeless, and stupid I was? That didn't happen. A new thought was freeing and comforting to me: I wasn't in danger because someone knew.

Feeling encouraged by the end of this visit, I asked if she knew of any good therapists. Having recently moved to a new state,

I viewed this as a good time to take advantage of a clean slate. I kept thinking about the decision I made when I'd said to God: "Fine, if others know about this, fine." My actions had yet to show I meant this decision. A few previous, unsuccessful bouts with disclosure left me feeling very reluctant and gun-shy. To say that I had trust issues would be an understatement; trust issues were, indeed, added to my "pile of issues." I had to deal with all of them though.

"He who covers his sins will not prosper,
But whoever confesses and forsakes them
will have mercy."
—Proverbs 28:13

My first unsuccessful disclosure attempt had been with my roommates during my sophomore year of college. As they became more frustrated with my erratic behavior, they enlisted help from my guidance counselor, the former nun, and another counselor. The four of them then "ganged up" on me. The second counselor contacted me, informing me that my roommates had set up a meeting with me. My attendance was strongly encouraged. With everything that had occurred that year, I didn't think they wanted to discuss the apartment decor. Cornered, with no way out, I had no choice but to participate in this meeting.

When the meeting finally took place, it felt like an ambush. We met in one of the college boardrooms, and even the seating arrangement singled me out. I sat alone at the end of the long table. My two roommates and the counselors sat on the opposite end of the long table. I'm not sure if this was an intentional battle plan, but I did feel like I was in a war. The four expressed concern for me, and my roommates confronted me about my behaviors. I was asked to seek professional help, which the school could provide for me. I reluctantly admitted what I had done and agreed to seek treatment. I took some comfort in knowing that I wouldn't have to deal with this for very long. This meeting occurred in March. I only had two months to go before transferring to another school the following year.

At that time I went to therapy only because I had to go, not because I wanted to go. In my opinion, eating disorder sufferers will go along with the flow because of their own need to avoid confrontation and conflict of any sort. But make no mistake about it, their will can be strong and their personal agendas can be firmly in place. I went to only two sessions with my appointed counselor. We barely scratched the surface of things. She weighed me, she had me draw a self-portrait showing how I saw myself, and we started talking about family issues related to my mother and father. I thought to myself the whole time, "I just need to make it to May, then I'm out of here!" After those two sessions, I canceled any other appointments with her through the month of May. I was "free" once again.

But this experience taught me something: maybe I *could* tell someone. This was a good three years before my "faithquake decision" and my search for God, but it did show me that I could survive someone knowing about my problem.

I had managed to make it through my college years without telling anyone. I even avoided dating because of one incident that was too close for comfort. I certainly couldn't let college guys know about this. I didn't want to take any chances.

As far as I was concerned, disclosing my eating track record would completely snuff out any chance I had with the opposite sex. How could they still view me as remotely attractive or worthwhile? I had a deep need to be pleasing, to show no signs of the trouble that these eating disorders represented. So I was the "cheap date" whenever I'd go out to dinner with someone. At most, I'd have just a salad. But usually, I'd just order a diet soft drink, and I'd never be very hungry, of course, whether I was or not.

Question: Do you feel uncomfortable eating in front of the opposite sex?

My "too close for comfort" date occurred late during my senior year of high school when I went on a casual date with a friend I'll call Tim.

We had been friends for a while, so I was surprised when he began flirting with me. At this time, I was at about 145–150 pounds, and in my mind, I was too large to receive attention, flirtation, or love. On one hand, I soaked his attention up. I was dehydrated for it, and it felt so wonderful to believe, even for a second, that he meant what he was saying to me. On the other hand, I had extreme difficulty in believing him. I kept waiting for the punch line, the joke, the laugh at my expense to happen. It didn't happen.

We went to dinner after classes one night. Of course, I was on a diet and ordered just a diet soft drink. He ordered a full meal. When our order came, he remarked jokingly, "You don't have one of those eating disorders like anorexia or bulimia, do you?" I was stunned. I quickly gathered whatever composure I could and did my usual denial. I laughed, going along with the joke. But it hurt me. I felt like my cheeks were two erupting volcanoes. I prayed that Tim wouldn't see this reaction. I tried to make sure my clammy hands weren't shaking too much when I picked up my drink to take a sip. Needless to say, this was our last date. The wall of protection grew higher and thicker. I distanced myself from him. I thought I was safe again, far away from any really close relationship. I was determined to avoid ever being more than "just friends" with any guy. Despite all of my notions, my attempts, and agendas, even this would gradually change.

"But we all, with unveiled face,
beholding as in a mirror the glory of the Lord,
are being transformed into the same image
from glory to glory,
just as by the Spirit of the Lord."
—2 Corinthians 3:18

Although I was craving love, I was determined to avoid it. I'd seen unhealthy relationships galore. I'd focused my life on achievement, convincing myself that the goals, awards, and prizes would be more than enough for me. And besides, college was demanding enough; I didn't need any more hassle. Still, I couldn't deny, I *did* want that hassle.

In college, I was pursuing a theater degree. My best performances weren't on the stage, but in my everyday life, protecting my secrets. Acting, lying—what's the difference, anyway? It was through theater that I met Russell, the first guy that I couldn't push away.

He was there for me.

I met Russell when I transferred schools. We were both theater students and met in the college drama department when I was a junior. We stayed on friendly, acquaintance-level terms through my graduation. He was sweet to me and possessed a dry sense of humor. It made for supportive, interesting, and funny conversations. Still, I looked at him the way I looked at other guys: a nice friend, but still someone who must never know all of my ugly weaknesses.

Even though we didn't start dating until after I graduated, our friendship was gradually changing while I was still in school. During my senior year of college, he was very thoughtful. For example, on Valentine's Day, he stopped by my dorm room. Of course, I had been on my stair stepper for hours and wouldn't come to the door. I kept yelling over the music, "I'm not done yet!" He waited as long as he could, but eventually he had to leave for work. When I finally finished my routine, I got my stuff together and headed for the dorm showers. When I opened my door, there was an overwhelmingly huge bouquet of balloons and a card. He had waited for at least a half hour for me, just to give me this sweet gift. All I said to him was, "I'm not done yet." I felt like the biggest jerk in the world.

When we did start to date and fall in love, I added new fears to my already long list. The prospect of someone being close enough to truly know me was scary. I knew that, sooner or later, I would have to tell him the ugly truth about myself.

Moving from dating to engagement was difficult for me. I had yet to tell him any of what I'd experienced, and I felt more and more guilty about lying to him. Every time we went out to eat, I'd pretend not to have issues with food and weight. I hated feeling like a liar, but I was scared that he'd reject me if he knew the truth. What man, in his right mind, looks for all of this mess in a mate? I knew when I told him that he wouldn't want me anymore. It bothered me constantly. He sensed something was wrong, of course, and asked me about it. *What do I tell him?* I couldn't begin to imagine.

Question: Do you withhold truth from those you love? How does it make you feel?

As we prepared for our wedding, I finally mentioned to him that I had a secret I wasn't ready to share with him yet. Of course, he was curious and wanted to know right then and there, but he displayed patient understanding. He told me that he loved me and that it didn't matter what it was. He didn't pressure me to tell him. He knew there was a secret and left it at that. Even though his response helped me feel freer and safer, I still felt guilt pulling at me. I began wanting to tell him. After all, he'd been so incredible with everything else I'd told him. He knew about my family secrets. He knew all about my weaknesses aside from the eating disorders. He knew about all that yet still chose to love me. But I kept thinking, *Don't press your luck*.

Remember the bridesmaid dress story from my cousin's wedding? Well, when it was my own wedding, multiply those insecurities and feelings by a thousand. The wedding dress alone was enough of a challenge. However, this time I wasn't able to go to extremes to lose weight for the wedding. Physically, there wasn't any way that I could reach that low weight from years earlier. It was a gift, though, that for the first time in a long time, I weighed a relatively normal 125 pounds on my wedding day. I was thankful for that.

I don't endorse my secrecy from my husband. I believe it is vital any young woman suffering from eating disorders be honest and forthcoming with her future husband. Marriage is a holy covenant and a serious commitment, and I believe you need to share all of the truth. Even now, I now look back and often wonder how many tears, how many problems, and how much pain I could have avoided if I just simply told him.

The time for truth came a couple of weeks after we were married. It was our first Thanksgiving together, and we had been married for only 12 days. I was still feeling relieved that I made it through the nuptials. Russ and I did the cutesy newly-wed couple "this is the first mashed potatoes we've made together" and "this is our first stuffing and cranberry sauce" thing. We both ate our holiday feast, and I tried not to think about all of the calories.

True to form, however, I proceeded to exercise after the meal, trying to burn off "the damage." Russell thought this was strange and unnecessary; it was a holiday, after all. He told me to just relax and enjoy the day. I, of course, repeatedly told him that I couldn't until I'd exercised. The conversation continued while I was on the stair stepper for two hours. But I saw a new look on his face: hurt. I was forfeiting my time with him, my brand-new husband, to climb steps that weren't going any-where. I was so tired of keeping this secret, and I wanted to explain myself so badly to him. The only way I could explain it was to tell him the whole story from the beginning. First, I played an alternative rock song, an anthem, a coping mecha-nism for me to deal with the eating disorders. It was an angry loud song of rage, and I thought that it would tell him clearly what I'd been through. It didn't. He didn't understand it. I took a deep breath, realizing, *No, Sheryle, the song isn't going to tell him. You are.* And so I did.

And the worst didn't happen. He didn't leave me, throw me out in the street, call me worthless, and tell me how much he hated me. No. He looked at me and asked, "This is the big secret?" He hugged me, told me he loved me, and told me I was beautiful. I didn't have to lie, hide, and pretend anymore in front of the man I loved. I felt a little freer. The truth really does set you free. And in telling him, once again, I discovered, the worst did not happen.

Since then, Russell has been an incredible support to me as I've continued my path in dealing with my food, weight, and body issues. It sounds so cliché, but it's true: He loves me just as I am. Does that sound a little too much like a fairy tale to be believed? Believe me, we've gone through less-than-fairy-tale moments, and those less-than-fairy-tale moments led me to yet another disclosure, the disclosure I briefly mentioned at the beginning of this chapter. I needed to seek professional help.

A **Prayer** to Rise

Father, I come to You in the name of Jesus, asking for help in my life. Thank You, Lord, that You know everything about me and that I am safe confessing anything and everything to You.

Lord, help me to be brave, to let others know what is going on with me. You know I've lived in secrecy and lies, protecting myself for so long. Forgive me for that. I am now finding out, however, that secrecy and lies are not protection, but confinement instead. I turn to You now, and I ask for help, guidance, and wisdom to let others know the truth about me.

This is a big step for me, Lord. I ask for love, acceptance, support, and encouragement from others to be the response to my disclosure. I recognize that this may not always be the response I receive. Therefore, I ask for grace, comfort, and forgiveness that can come only from You to help me through these challenging experiences.

Thank you, Lord that the truth is setting me free **(John 8:32),** and I don't need to be afraid. I only need to trust in You. I do this now by faith. In Jesus's name, I pray. Amen.

Journaling Section
To Help You **Work Through** Your Thoughts

Are you afraid to have people know "the real you"? Why?

_____

_____

_____

_____

_____

_____

_____

How do you feel about dating and relationships with the opposite sex? How do you eat when you're with someone of the opposite sex?

_____

_____

_____

_____

_____

_____

Describe your relationship with your family members. How do you feel about them? What can you do to change those relationships, if needed?

_____

_____

_____

_____

_____

_____

_____

How do family members feel about your behaviors concerning dieting, food, and weight?

_____

_____

_____

_____

_____

_____

_____

Who have you told the truth about your food and weight issues?

_____

_____

_____

_____

_____

_____

How do you feel about having them know this about you?

_____

_____

_____

_____

_____

_____

_____

Scriptures to Consider

Jeremiah 30:17   2 Corinthians 3:18
Proverbs 28:13

When You Decide to Tell Someone
(Author's Personal Experience)

- Tell someone you trust and feel comfortable talking with, such as a pastor, counselor, family member, or friend.
- Don't dwell on their anticipated reaction. They may or may not receive the disclosure well. It can be a difficult thing for someone to handle. Remember that.
- Keep the disclosure honest, simple, and to the point: "I have an eating disorder, and I need your help."
- Be honest and open with where you are now and what you are doing.
- If it helps make things easier, give the person a book on the eating disorder, or write a letter to explain your situation and answer any questions they may have.
- Don't take their reactions personally. You are not to blame if they don't take the news well.
- Whenever possible, choose professional help to be a part of your support system. A pastor or counselor familiar with the treatment of eating disorders can help in your treatment.
- Surround yourself with a positive group of supporters who desire to love and encourage you.
- Be patient with yourself and with others during this process. It takes time.
- Be proud of yourself for this step! It shows tremendous courage on your part.

Chapter Eight

Wounds to Scars

Salt in the Wound

The little girl
discovered salt
as it fell from her tears,
Salt in the wound,
She had to feel it
instead of letting it
preserve
the hurt,
The little girl
needed to decide
what would live
and what would die
to her,
She had to cry
tears of pain,
tears of truth
in order
to feel
better,
Salt in the wound,
Painful
Truthful
Hurt,
She had to live through it,

and then
let it die,
Only then
could God begin
to heal her,
as God
started turning wounds
into scars.

ThinEnough

Eating disorders are not about food. Food is just the vehicle; the unsuccessful method used to process and express whatever pain, whatever issues are going on already. And once that vehicle, that method, is removed from the equation, there leaves a gap awaiting its replacement.

Because I was gradually progressing in a healthier diet and exercise routine, I soon began to see that food really wasn't the problem at all. I still had problems and issues that wouldn't go away. I was struggling with depression, despair, and at the ugly root of it all, rage. Good nutrition and proper exercise have a lot to offer toward improving the quality of one's life. They cannot, however, fully deal with "unfinished business." Only God can do that. And it seemed like that's what He was gently, but firmly, doing for me.

I didn't know what to do with all of the lingering issues from my past. I had faced my addiction to food, to approval, to control. I could accept that. But another addiction—anger—proved more difficult to accept.

Question: Do you struggle with anger directed toward yourself or others?

Me, angry? At first, I thought it was ridiculous. After all, I was raised to be the "good girl," who never became upset. Sugar and spice and everything nice, right? No, I didn't have an anger problem. And I guess there was a part of me that didn't see it as even possible for girls to be capable of anger. I looked at how the women in my family lived. I saw how they couldn't and wouldn't disagree with anyone, especially their husbands. They chose, instead, to stuff all of their pain down and pretend that it didn't exist. I learned how to do that as well. It's a dangerous volcano, however, living this way. Sooner or later, on somebody or another, you will erupt. And that's what I did.

My anger was mostly aimed at my father. As far as I was concerned, he was to blame! I felt abandoned, orphaned, and left alone by my father. I was saddled with problems that belonged to my parents and not to me. I wondered if a close, loving relationship with him would have prevented all my mistakes. My running thought became, "This would not have happened if my daddy loved me." This sense of injustice, of rejection, of being wronged became the filter through which I viewed everything in life.

I *was* mad. I wanted explanations; I wanted answers! No one around me, however, could give me those answers. And God didn't seem to be clueing me in, either. So I cried and screamed frustrated tears, ranting within myself about how unfair it was that other girls got to have loving fathers. Other girls got the chance to be "daddy's girl." Why not me?

As a way of dealing with my demons, I directed a lot of my pain into writing. I was part of a drama troupe that wrote and performed their own pieces, and it became a release valve for me. As an attempt to deal with my frustration and pain about the whole situation, I wrote a spiteful short dramatic piece entitled *Daddy's Girl*.

With my *Daddy's Girl* drama, I went for as much of the murky girl, seething, and violent expression of pain I could get (without committing a felony). My pen was my weapon. I felt vindicated each time it was performed. I would not act out any of the roles written. Instead, I passed it on to fully capable divas and drama queens, knowing they'd take it to my desired extreme. I loved watching the shock and the gasps of the crowd as my story made them uncomfortable. I was high from this revenge, but the feeling never lasted. Instead, what remained was pain from the hollow reminder of what I didn't have and sheer desperation from sinking so low with revenge. The audience went home; I went home. Revenge didn't change matters any. I still wanted to be "daddy's little girl."

> *"Beloved, do not avenge yourselves,*
> *but rather give place to wrath;*
> *for it is written, 'Vengeance is Mine,*
> *I will repay,' says the Lord.*
> *'Therefore if your enemy hungers, feed him;*
> *If he thirsts, give him a drink.'"*
> *—Romans 12:19–20*

I took most of my frustration and anger out on my husband. He was safe for me, and since we lived far away from my parents, he was the only family I had. Suddenly, anything he did that remotely resembled my father's behavior became fair game. Things that attracted me to Russell began to change in my eyes. My husband's quick wit? I began to see it as a personal attack. His understanding nature? I saw it as him patronizing me. On and on and on…. I was suppressing so much anger. I thought it was clear-cut: My father caused all of this pain, and I was left to deal with the wreckage. I'd constantly scream within myself, "It's not fair!" Maybe I was only a pathetic, low self-esteem, eating disorder, basket-case poster girl after all!

Like so many times before, I thought I could run away from who I was. Russell and I made the move from Minnesota to

Oregon, but a new state doesn't necessarily guarantee a new life. All of my issues packed their bags as well.

During this move I started feeling tired and ill. I thought it was just the stress of the move, but it persisted even when we were settled. I went to see a naturopathic doctor for answers. She first treated me physically and was a compassionate, unshakable sounding board for the disclosure of my eating disorder history. However, she then allowed for it to be "my idea" to seek professional help, which was incredibly freeing, empowering for me. Eating disorder sufferers oftentimes feel that they have no choice in areas of their own lives. So they'll take control in any way they can get it. When I made this choice to seek help, I felt that I didn't have anything to lose. I was an adult, far away from the threat of my parents and school. And let's face it, I wasn't happy and I wanted to deal with all these issues. If it wasn't about the food, then what *was* it about?

From the list of referrals, I chose a doctor I'll call Dr. Fay. I was nervous about the initial consultation. This was the most active I'd ever been in admitting the truth about what I'd gone through. I had only willingly disclosed my history to Russell and my physician. When others intervened, there was an element of comfort in knowing that I could deny and wiggle my way out of it. However, initiating help myself meant that there was no turning back once I stated the truth.

When I met with Dr. Fay for the consultation, I immediately noticed the box of tissues on the table. I had been trying to steel myself, toughen up enough so that I wouldn't cry. Crying, for me, was a sign of weakness. I kept trying to convince myself that this pursuit of therapy was a sign of strength instead. I repeatedly told myself to buck up. However, despite all of my determination, I had a big crying session after the initial contract and methodology information. "Great first impression, Sheryle," I thought. I didn't quite appreciate the absurdity of it all. Typical me: I wanted to impress my therapist? Please! But I did feel better after the session. I saw the eating disorder issue as a giant balloon. Little by little, as I told the truth to more people, I was deflating it.

For the record, I want to state that Dr. Fay, however excellent a therapist, was a secular therapist. While matters of God and faith did pop up occasionally, she remained neutral with the subject of Christianity. Looking back on it, I would ideally choose a Christian counselor. So many of life's issues are caught up in guilt, sin, God's acceptance, love, and forgiveness. So much empowerment comes from our connecting with the Holy Spirit. These were areas that Dr. Fay had no expertise in.

Without treatment, up to 20 percent of people with serious eating disorders die. With treatment, that number falls to 2–3 percent. With treatment, about 60 percent of people with eating disorders recover. In spite of treatment, about 20 percent of people with eating disorders make only partial recoveries. The remaining 20 percent do not improve, even with treatment. Please note: The study of eating disorders is a relatively new field. We have no good information on the long-term recovery process. We do know that recovery usually takes a long time, perhaps on average three to five years of slow progress that includes starts, stops, slides backward, and ultimately, movement in the direction of mental and physical health.

ANRED, "Statistics: How Many People Have Eating Disorders?" http://www.anred.com/stats.html. Used with permission.

So Dr. Fay and I proceeded with my weekly sessions. I was surprised to discover that the eating disorders rarely came up as topics of conversation. Instead, we focused on my relationship to my father. "A-ha!" I thought, "This was his fault, after all." I was ready for some heavy-duty blaming directed right at him. My first few sessions were angry rants about how he did this and how he said that, and so on. But as time progressed, I started to change my view of him.

During this time, my father's health was deteriorating. As Mom shared the signs of his failing health with me, my attitude changed. Growing up, there was a time when I hated my father and wished he was dead. I couldn't wait for the day when he died, letting Mom and me go. But now, he wasn't the indestructible force I once knew. All I could now feel was pity. What was going on here?

Another change that was taking place was a change in my writing style. For the longest time, writing had been my venting weapon. I'd write dark, brooding moody poems and plays of revenge. I'd go on a verbal tirade, showing him—showing *someone* that I was nobody's victim, nobody's fool! But I was miserable and stifled creatively the whole time. I felt the urge to write happier, lighter things. Who, me? Write about puppies and kittens and rainbows? Only if the rainbows are brutally killing the puppies and kittens. But I couldn't get it out of my head. So, to humor God or myself or whomever, I started writing more inspirational stuff. "Happier" is the puppy/kitten domain. "Inspirational" seemed to me to be more real. I started having more creative bursts. I was even happier as I started to believe my own writing.

God wasn't just dealing with one area in my life. He works on the entire person. Everything in each individual's life is interconnected. So when God is fixing me through therapy, diet, and exercise, He's also fixing my attitudes, emotions, and feelings. I soon found myself turning to the Bible for inspiration. I was continuing to heal as I read, wrote, and found the Father I'd always wanted, but never had. When the revelation about Jairus's daughter and my rededication happened years earlier, I was initially so focused on Jesus, I forgot there was a Father God in the picture as well. But as I read and wrote, I found myself writing to God, my Father. Eventually, all I was writing was faith-based, Word-based, inspirational stuff. I wasn't so harsh about life anymore. I wanted revenge less and peaceful restoration more. This attitude went beyond my passion for writing. It started extending into my life as well.

Question: Do you struggle with issues of forgiveness?

One of the main realizations I gained about my father through therapy was that he was a person, too. He wasn't my enemy, a villain, or a monster. He was a man. My father was 49 years old when I was born, and fatherhood, I'm sure, was an unexpected new role for him. Having never been parented in a nurturing home himself, he wasn't equipped to give me that atmosphere of unconditional support and love. As I pondered this, I decided to go through some photographs. My dad, reclusive in nature, is pretty camera-shy, and there aren't a lot of pictures of him. But there is one rare one of him as a child no more than six years old. He's sitting on some farm equipment, next to one of his brothers. As I looked at this picture, it hit me: My dad was once a child.

As I stared at this image, at this little boy with the mop head of bangs, wearing overalls and no shoes, I couldn't hate him. I couldn't hate a little boy; I couldn't hate a child. I couldn't hate *God's* child. Instead, I found myself wanting to connect with him somehow. I was nowhere near direct communication. I hadn't spoken to him or seen him in years. But I wanted to touch him; I wanted to reach him somehow. The only way I knew how to physically touch him was to draw him. I drew the little boy.

It sounds too simple, but it did help. It didn't matter what hurtful things he'd said to me some 50 years after that photo was taken. He was a little boy "subject" now, and I could choose to draw him any way I decided. After drawing him as this innocent little boy, I didn't want to return to the way I'd drawn him before. Hating someone and refusing to forgive them takes a lot of energy. I was tired, and I didn't want to do it anymore.

I had a revelation about forgiveness. For my entire life, I'd viewed forgiveness as something that denied the occurrence of a wrong. He hurt me, and I didn't want anyone, especially him, telling me otherwise. But forgiveness, I was finding out, wasn't denying a wrong. It was just adding God's healing power to that wrong. And I needed forgiveness just as much as my father did

"And whenever you stand praying, if you have anything against anyone, forgive him, that your Father in heaven may also forgive you your trespasses."
—Jesus, in Mark 11:25

The buzz of the new millennium was in the air. Everyone was thinking of starting new, starting again. Could it apply to the relationship with my dad? I saw this as a perfect opportunity to try, at least. So I wrote my dad a New Year's card, thanking him for everything he'd been and done for me. I also asked for his forgiveness, for hurting him in the past. And I told him I hoped we could become closer in the new year and the new millennium. I signed it "I love you, Sheryle." That was probably the most difficult thing I have ever written. I honestly didn't even know if I really meant it. But I did start wanting to mean it. I felt better after writing it. I decided to forgive him—even if that meant the feelings would come later. I waited. His move, right?

Question: Do you need to forgive someone for your own sake?

Dr. Fay applauded my efforts, while cautioning me at the same time. She didn't want me getting my hopes up too high. Indeed, I might not get the desired result, not that I knew what that would be. But writing and sending this card, for now, was enough.

Once Dr. Fay and I worked through my relationship with my dad, I thought I had all of my issues wrapped up. Not quite. I still had one parent to go.

My mother: My best friend? My ally? My enemy? Who was she to me? Once I felt a little more at ease with my father, Dr. Fay wanted to delve into the wonderful world of mother/daughter relationships. I knew that I had "issues" with Mom, of course, but I honestly thought they were under control. I came to therapy to deal with my dad. Mom wasn't the problem. I knew she loved me. She'd sacrificed so much of her life for me. I didn't have *that* much of a problem with her, did I?

Dr. Fay asked me about how well I got along with her lately. I told her that we talked on the phone regularly. At this point, she asked me about the move from Minnesota to Oregon. How did my mother feel about it? Honestly, Mom wasn't happy about me moving so far away. She had always talked about all of the plans that "we" were going to make, all of the things "we" were going to do. No matter what I wanted to do, it was always a "team" thing with her. Her dreams always included me, and my dreams should always, therefore, include her: together forever.

Growing up in a sheltered environment, college offered my first timid steps away from her world. I discovered that I loved my freedom. Despite the fact that my behaviors were far from healthy in college, I certainly didn't want to go back to that cage. I was free. I was living my life, or so I thought. Even if my eating disorders became my life, at least they were mine, not hers, and certainly not "ours." No, Mom, this belonged to me!

So the tug of war ensued. The more I wanted to run away from home, the more she wanted to keep me there. I resented that greatly. She, of all people, knew that dysfunctional situation and how stifling it was. Wouldn't she want me free and happy? That's what she always said, but then she would turn around and encourage "our dreams and plans" again, which were close to home, while discouraging mine, which were further away.

I felt like I had two extremes going on here. My father didn't want me at all, and my mother wanted me too much. Mother bashing became the new focus of my sessions with Dr. Fay. I began to wonder if my father's lack of involvement in my life was not because he wasn't interested in me, but rather because he simply didn't see any room for himself in my life. I suddenly found myself embittered toward my mother. Had she stolen my father from me in order to have more of me for herself? I started to feel like I had issues with the wrong parent. I felt angry, confused. Who do I blame?

ThinEnough

I wanted a scapegoat. None of this was making sense. Food wasn't my enemy? My father wasn't my enemy? It had to be Mom then, right? All I was left with was more questions and more pain. I felt like, once again, I wasn't getting any better, only angrier and more wrong. Basically, I lived a temper tantrum 27 years in the making.

Question: Do you feel the need for a scapegoat?

While still stewing in my anger toward my mother, I did get feedback from my father regarding the New Year's card. It wasn't directly from him, but, in one of my conversations with my mother (I was still talking to her), I found out that he read it silently to himself and smiled. According to my mother, he kept it by his chair and looked at it from time to time. Mom told me she thought it made him happy. I was tempted to feel slighted by his easy happiness here, but I couldn't hate him anymore.

More and more of my sessions were spent crying. I didn't know what to make of this. What I was doing here? Accepting? Grieving? Maybe I wasn't crying or grieving specifically for my father or mother. Maybe I wasn't even crying for myself. Maybe I was grieving instead for the situation, not just what happened to me, but what happened to all of us.

We all bought into our "should" lives: This is the way "life should be." When life didn't happen that way for any of us, we each turned to the God substitute of our choice. My dad's substitute was work and money. My mother's substitute was being the peacekeeping wife and mother. And me? Well, I chose self-destruction and feelings of worthlessness and secrecy. There you have it: our idols. Each of us, in our own way rejected and disobeyed God. Each of us, not just me, was God's wounded child who needed to forgive and be forgiven.

I couldn't control what my parents or anyone else did, but I could control my actions. I chose to let God help me forgive them. I accepted the fact that this is a process. I believe they call it "life." I wanted to get on with mine.

Did I mention all of this to Dr. Fay? No. Truth be told, as I was nearing the completion of one year of therapy, I was having mixed feelings. Although I did feel like I made progress in dealing with disclosure issues of honesty, safety, and trust (I even let my mother in on "the secret" that I was going to therapy), I still felt restless, especially spiritually. Dr. Fay, as wonderful as she was, still wasn't providing me with the answers that I needed. I felt like she had taken me only so far on my pathway. God had to pick up fully from there.

And I needed some semblance of roots in my life. Having lived in Oregon for about a year, I still didn't feel like I was home. I felt like I should move away from this therapy, as helpful as it was, and move closer to an actual church, with actual people. I needed to go from man's help to God's help. For so long, I had desired to belong to a family, to a community. I wanted to be a part of who God was and where He hung out.

In my pursuit of this community, I proceeded to "church hop," bouncing from one church to the next. It was a frustrating process. I didn't feel like I belonged. I had voluntarily made my choice to leave this safety net of my secular therapy for that of a more godly approach. Was this my result? Was I sentenced to unending, nose-pressed-up-against-the-glass experiences even here, where I should be most accepted?

As seems to be God's way with me, things were changing gradually. I was in need of patience. But the cat was a little more out of the bag, and I was a little more out of my painful cage.

A **Prayer** to Rise

Father, I come to You in the name of Jesus, asking for help in my life. Thank You, Lord, that You are my healer, no matter how deep the hurt or pain.

I ask You, Lord, for healing for every part of me: spirit, emotions, body. You know those wounds that are so deep nothing and no one else can reach them. Only You, Lord, can heal, and I ask You, Lord, to heal me now.

Thank You for the healing that comes from the passage of time, for healing that comes from Your compassionate people, and for healing that comes from reading and experiencing Your Word in my life. Continue, Lord, to work Your restoration, whatever form that healing may be. I trust You, in Your love and wisdom, to do only what's best for me.

Thank You for Your promise. Your Word tells me that You have heard my prayer and You have seen my tears, and You surely will heal me **(2 Kings 20:5)**. I receive this healing Word now and I thank You for it. In Jesus's name, I pray. Amen.

Journaling Section

To Help You **Work Through** Your Thoughts

What anger do you have toward yourself? Toward others?
Toward God?

_____

_____

_____

_____

_____

_____

What would you like to tell yourself, others, God, if you
knew it was safe to do so?

_____

_____

_____

_____

_____

ThinEnough

How do you feel about therapy/counseling?

_____

_____

_____

_____

_____

_____

Is there someone you need to forgive?

_____

_____

_____

_____

In what ways do you need to be forgiven?

_____

_____

_____

_____

_____

What do you think will happen if you forgive or ask for forgiveness?

_____

_____

_____

_____

_____

_____

How does anger/lack of forgiveness affect your eating habits and the way you view yourself?

_____

_____

_____

_____

_____

_____

Scriptures to Consider

Romans 12:19   2 Kings 20:5

Mark 11:25

Questions to Ask When Seeking Treatment

- What can I expect to happen during sessions?
- How much experience have you had working with people who have eating disorders?
- Tell me about your training, education, and licenses.
- How long do you think treatment will take?
- How often will we meet?
- If I think I need to, can I call you between sessions?
- What are your thoughts about using medications in the treatment of eating disorders?
- Could I be put in a hospital against my will? (This is a common fear. Get the facts at the beginning so you will know what to expect.)
- How much do sessions cost? Do you take insurance? What if my insurance will not cover all the costs of treatment?
- If I don't think I'm improving fast enough, I may feel like either you or I am failing. What can I do if that happens? (Be sure to ask this one. Don't just drop out if you get discouraged. Overcoming "stuckness" in treatment is a major victory.)

ANRED, "Treatment and Recovery," http://www.anred.com/tx.html. Used with permission.

Family Intervention and Therapy

In order to help a person with an eating disorder:

- Feelings of intense guilt and anxiety must be addressed.
- Family must understand the danger of the disorder.
- Family members must acknowledge their collaboration in the patient's illness.
- Appropriate interpersonal boundaries need to be established.
- Needs and feelings of the patient must be recognized, accepted, and articulated.
- Sense of self should be separate from parents, especially that of mother and daughter.

Adapted from Ohio State University FactSheet, "Eating Disorders Awareness: Emotional Issues Involved With Eating Disorders," http://ohioline.osu.edu/ed-fact/1005.html.

Chapter Nine

The Relearning Process

Suddenly (from Gradually)

Suddenly
From gradually
the mirror looked different
as the little girl caught a glimpse
Different
somehow
Was it a trick?
An illusion?
Fun house torture played upon her?
Or was it
Maybe
Reality
Suddenly
From gradually
The little girl started seeing
herself
differently
Maybe
She wasn't so bad
after all
She wondered
if she could call
her body

Herself
okay
Suddenly
From gradually
mirror
became different
Was it the mirror?
Or was it herself
somehow
Suddenly
The gradually
gave way
and what seemed to stay
was God
God loving her
She wasn't so bad
She was even okay
even
dare she say
pretty?
Suddenly
God changed the mirror
God changed her
to help her see
The beloved image
God's
love
envisioned her
created her
to be.

Being the intense, dramatic person I can sometimes be, I often find myself waiting for the big "ta-da" moments to show up. And God is definitely a "ta-da" kind of God, but I believe that most of my breakthroughs were more subtle and gradual. He graciously started giving me encouraging, subtle "ta-da" miracles. And through it all, He has been—and still is—very patient with me.

I did my initial "church hopping" still within the boundaries of my denominational background though, convincing myself that eventually I'd find the right church. I was growing restless and frustrated each time I sat in the back row of another church, hoping that maybe this one was it. I had some close calls. I'd spoken to pastors, filled out visitor forms, but situations didn't pan out in the end. Why weren't they panning out? With no answer, I'd hop to another church.

The churches I was hopping to were getting less traditional. I began to think about going outside of my denominational pool. Yes, color outside of the lines! This seemed to be a kooky idea to me. In my family, you stayed within your denominational walls. You didn't go traipsing into unknown territory. Oh, the scandal it raised within our family if and when someone should convert to another system. But God was leading me in another direction. (I'm not saying that God will always lead you away from your denomination; I'm just saying that's how it happened for me.)

Living in Portland, still getting used to the city, I passed a local Christian church one day on my way home. A thought popped into my head: *Give this one a try*. I argued with the thought. But faced with the frustrated dead end "searches for churches" so far, I agreed to at least see what it was about.

I went that Sunday, and this place was different! The first thing that struck me was how big and bright it was. What next hit me was the choir. A sucker for music, I was hooked. Something special was going on here. They were dancing and swaying to the infectious worship songs. And yes, they were smiling and having fun. Everyone looked like they wanted to be there!

Question: Do you have a church community/family where you feel you belong?

I decided to do a trial period here, just to see if this was the place. It felt out of my comfort zone, but I also couldn't deny the exciting, dynamic energy of the place. So I kept coming. Weeks turned into months. The place's name was a part of the reason I stayed: New Beginnings. Does God have a sense of humor here, or what? After all, I'd always sought after the new start, the fresh beginning point.

I wasn't the only one with a story at this place. The pastors and congregation members alike seemed to all have their own stories. They weren't fairy-tale perfect stories, but rather accounts of God's miraculous deliverance and healing at work in their lives. For so long I'd viewed church people and pastors as untouched by weakness and folly. But now, I could take some comfort in knowing that there were others who had "been through stuff" as well.

> *"For all have sinned and fall short*
> *of the glory of God."*
> *—Romans 3:23*

I didn't exactly plunge into this new world. It was a gradual, slow process for me. But I continued going every Sunday, sitting in the ver-r-ry back row, close to the exits, while still possessing both the attitude *get in, get God, get out quickly* and the sense of not belonging. Weeks passed with me desiring to become a part of God's family, while hardly speaking to anyone at all. How's that for logic? While the mature adult in me recognized the need to take some risks and actually talk to someone—hey, maybe even be friendly—the little kid in me still put up her *I don't want to and you can't make me!* argument.

"A man who has friends must himself be friendly."
—Proverbs 18:24

God, however, made sure that it was different this time. People talked to me here, made me feel included. That was different; I was so used to being left alone. Initially, it was somewhat irritating to me to be "bothered" like this. But wait a minute, wasn't this what I wanted in the first place?

I was being tweaked. I believe the biblical term is "pruned." As I continued attending this church, I had more thoughts pop into my head, like "Why don't you..." followed then by a suggestion to talk to a person, hug a person, check out more information about this opportunity, event, etc. With each tweaking, coaxing question, I shot back my typical arguments about why I shouldn't. God is ver-r-ry patient. Did I mention already?

I signed up for a seminar about discovering your spiritual gifts. It sounded intriguing. I was ready for the information. The class was informative, interesting, just what I had counted on. But I hadn't counted on gaining more than information. As I looked for a place to sit, a woman started talking with me. She asked if we could sit together and I agreed. She was sweet, loving, and a very chatty Cathy, but she was real. And when the class was over, she wanted to stay in touch. And there you have it: friendship—even for this loner. Her friendship was the unexpected gift that I came away with that day.

"God sets the solitary in families."
—Psalm 68:6

This seemed to me to be God's method of bringing people to me. I'd sign up to attend classes or join a small group study in someone's house, with the sole objective of learning or achieving something, and come away from the experience actually *knowing* someone. And knowing people soon led to hugging people. Yes, I'd found myself becoming one of those huggers, milling around happily in the church beehive. I was suspicious about this whole thing here. I wondered what was going on, quite frankly, as the "huggy" experiences, the warm fuzzy experiences with people started happening more and more. It was like someone (God?) was deliberately placing a "Hug me" sign on me. And, as awkward as it felt, I loved it. I loved being loved. I loved learning how to be loved.

For most people, the issue of dealing and communicating with other people on a daily basis is not an earth-shattering revelation. But I had allowed my world to become so small, so isolated, due in large part to my controlling need for self-protection. That left little room for anyone to get into my life.

But now, desiring change and a closer relationship with God, I had to get used to people again. I had to get used to knowing people and being known by them.

As I was getting to know more people, I started taking more risks. I had more support, prayers, and cheerleading from others than I'd ever experienced before in my life. I'd move step by step, it seemed, finding myself stepping into more foreign territory, more questions. Nowhere was this more evident than with one of the best gifts God has given me: an internship program within the church. Within the program, a small group of people focused on both developing their walk with God and serving the Lord through its volunteer service component. Both of these objectives would impact me profoundly and draw me closer to experiencing more of God's love.

"Your ears shall hear a word behind you,
saying, 'This is the way, walk in it,'
Whenever you turn to the right hand
Or whenever you turn to the left.'"
—Isaiah 30:21

Here's where God used the tactic "Let her feel loved, loved, loved." This went beyond the incredible love I'd experienced just through Sunday services. With this group of fellow God-seekers, everything was amplified, including that whole "God's family" thing. And I was in need of learning how to become a part of God's family.

*"I will instruct you and teach you
in the way you should go;
I will guide you with My eye."*
—Psalm 32:8

Person after person conveyed the message to me that I belonged. Terms of endearment were commonplace for me now, although it took (and still takes) some getting used to. I was called "honey/sweetie/dear/darling" more than I had ever experienced in my entire life. The impact of these simple words was huge. I was not used to being thought of in sweet, loving terms. I had to practice hearing, believing, and accepting these things being said to and about me. I had to, in short, practice being loved by God. It's a bit mind-blowing to sit and think that maybe God Himself thinks of us in terms of endearment. But, after all, at one time or another, most parents address their children by "honey" or "sweetie." Why not God, the ultimate loving Father? Whatever the reasoning behind it all, I couldn't deny how healed I was feeling—a little bit here, a little bit there.

*"Pleasant words are like a honeycomb,
Sweetness to the soul and health to the bones."*
—Proverbs 16:24

Then, God launched His next tactic: the let-her-experience-feeling-beautiful tactic. As it was getting a little easier for me to feel special, loved, and a sense of belonging, it was time for a physical self-image overhaul. I wasn't doing the roller-coaster thing anymore. I seemed to hang around the 120–130–pound range. This, in and of itself, meant a lot to me, not necessarily because those numbers had any magic to them, but rather because I didn't have to struggle to the death to keep them. Indeed, maybe this was, after all, what I was supposed to weigh. It was a weight that looked healthy on me, but more than that, it felt healthy on me. Now it was okay, acceptable; it even felt a little successful.

And during this time with the internship program, I had now become busier with other things other than weight and body issues. Disordered eating and image habits often consume and take over every part of life. But now, my life was being taken up more by God and the things of God. I didn't have the luxury any longer of obsessing about my looks—or for that matter, any other little thing about myself. I had stuff to do. It seemed to be ringing true, the whole thing about losing your life to save it (**Luke 9:23–24**). Yes, I was so much happier, so much freer, when it wasn't solely about me, me, and me. Last time I checked, "it" seemed to be about God.

"For where envy and self-seeking exist,
confusion and every evil thing will be there."
—James 3:16

And here's where a funny thing started happening. When I stopped thinking so much, obsessing so much about who

I was, what I looked like, I started getting more compliments and attention on my physical appearance. It was happening. And it wasn't even necessarily on my cute days either, those instances when you are "on." There were days when I felt I looked like Jabba the Hutt and was retaining water like Lake Erie. But those things, those "facts" didn't hold a candle to what God's Word said about me. Over and over again, I would read in the Bible about how God considered me to be **"beautiful,"** **"beloved."** (Check out the Song of Solomon here for this repetition of adjectives—a fantastic ego boost!) I was **"fearfully and wonderfully made" (Psalm 139:14).** Now, come on, did I really want to argue with all of that? Where the old me would have both argued that point and hidden away, refusing to face life and the world itself, I now had things to do that involved going about my Father's business.

"Delight yourself also in the LORD,
And He shall give you the desires of your heart."
—Psalm 37:4

As I was basking in this new life, I couldn't help but be reminded of years earlier when I'd craved and received attention and compliments. I didn't want to fall into the trap of being addicted to that praise. I wanted to be careful. But this time around, the attention became instead an open door for me to talk about God, not about me. People were asking me why I was so happy, why I was smiling, why I seemed different. All I had to do was tell them: God. In doing so, I received more than just the happy glow of a compliment from my appearance; I received an overwhelming peaceful contentment. As I was built up from each incident, I could feel myself glow. I was so happy with who I was becoming, valuable as God's child, not just for what I looked like. The compliments on my appearance were merely the icing on the cake. My identity was in God now.

I was relearning confidence, even in the midst of anxiety and fear. Through the internship's completion and through my continued volunteer work in the church, I found myself repeatedly asking God, "You want me to do *what*?" to the situations and opportunities that presented themselves to me. It all started with the copy machine. The copy machine, believe it or not, was something new to me. Initially, it seemed harmless enough: press a button and *voilà*! As I'd do more projects, requiring different things (heaven forbid, not two-sided, three-hole-punched copies, and on colored paper at that! No, please, not that! And enlarged to 125 percent, too? Oh, the horror!), I was getting more comfortable with being uncomfortable. I was getting more comfortable with doing tasks, without understanding absolutely everything in vivid detail as to why I was doing them in the first place. I was learning how to be capable—and how to trust God.

Question: Do you believe you have gifts to offer others that aren't related to your physical appearance?

I even found myself in situations where I was leading small groups of prayer and discussion. Hardly Billy Graham stadium-packed stuff, but practice in confidence nonetheless. Repeatedly I'd be placed in situations requiring management and delegation. No matter what the circumstance, God always helped me through. There were many times of crisis, when my first thought was to suck my thumb, but I didn't have that luxury. I did, however, have desperation for God, and He always came through. I had a lot of "Whew!" experiences, a lot of successes that He mercifully allowed me to experience. My confidence was growing, no doubt. I was feeling better about myself, my life, my relationship with God.

"Therefore do not cast away your confidence,
which has great reward.
For you have need of endurance,
so that after you have done the will of God,
you may receive the promise."
—Hebrews 10:35–36

So let's tally the results so far. God's giving me experiences in feeling special, in belonging, especially to a family, and in feeling beautiful. Was I destined to experience only warm fluffy, feel-good stuff? Well, not quite. Yes, God was building me up, restoring, repairing, and healing me. But I believe He had to get me to a point where I would feel a safety during the next challenging time.

Up until this point, I'd been riding this wave of reassuring love and support. I was in an ideal environment, surrounded by loving supportive people, receiving constant daily love lessons from them. If I had my way, I would have chosen to simply bask in that love constantly, soaking it up like a lizard soaking up the sun. But there was still more to God's love for me than basking.

*"Casting all your care upon Him,
for He cares for you."*
—1 Peter 5:7

*"Being confident of this very thing,
that He who has begun a good work in you
will complete it until the day of Jesus Christ."*
—Philippians 1:6

Criticism is bound to come, and I had to learn how to deal with it. For most of my life, I'd equated love with being perfect, being pleasing. Destructive criticism occurred in my past, hurting me, directly attacking me with such labels of "worthless" and "stupid." Now constructive criticism existed to help me. Just because I'd failed at doing something 100 percent perfectly did not mean that I was 100 percent worthless.

And I needed to learn that this part of the process, although not the most fun part, was not designed to make me feel like I was the most worthless, stupid person on the planet. Rather, it was also part of God's love. The old phrase "Love hurts" runs true.

While participating in the internship program, I held on to a bad habit of lurking behind a door anytime I needed to speak with someone in their office, instead of just confidently, calmly, and respectfully announcing my presence in an opened doorway. The behavior was, quite frankly, ridiculous, although I wasn't seeing it as being so at the time. One day, while I was working on a project in one pastor's office he called me on it. He stood in his own office doorway, announcing that he wanted to show me something. He then lurked behind the door, with just his eyeballs and nose sticking out from around the corner. That's what I look like, huh? Okay, point taken. He then showed me the correct, confident, nontimid approach.

> *"My son, do not despise the chastening of the LORD,*
> *Nor detest His correction;*
> *For whom the LORD loves He corrects,*
> *Just as a father the son in whom he delights."*
> *—Proverbs 3:11–12*

Elementary, yes, but this basic little thing represented a bigger key issue for me. A notorious "apologizer," I still conveyed a need to hide myself. Why was this happening? The location, the environment, the people were all different in my life. Why wasn't I? The answer that popped in my mind was, *Because you're not choosing to be.*

That stung! You mean to tell me that, in spite of all of the self-discovery, the information, the knowledge, and the wisdom I'd been given, I still wasn't "there"? I still wasn't "done"? I was beginning to feel hopeless again. Why was I experiencing this success and achievement, only to seemingly have it all come crashing down on me? Again, the key word, I came to find out, was *me.* Stubborn willed that I am by nature, I was still relying very much on my own strength, my own information, knowledge, wisdom, instead of God's. Indeed, I was leaning way too much on my own understanding.

"Trust in the LORD with all your heart,
And lean not on your own understanding;
In all your ways acknowledge Him,
And He shall direct your paths."
—Proverbs 3:5–6

Question: Do you feel solely responsible for fixing everything that's wrong?

The whole correction thing has taught me a lot about just how much I still argue with God about things, pointless as it is. I wanted to be "God's child" more than anything. I guess I had "childlike" and "childish" confused though. Childlike would have responded, "Yes, Lord, Your will be done; I trust You." Childish continually argued, "No! I don't want to! Mine! Mine! Mine!"

"Behold, happy is the man whom God corrects;
Therefore do not despise the chastening
of the Almighty."
—Job 5:17

"And by His stripes we are healed."
—*Isaiah 53:5*

Question: Do you believe that God can heal?

Over and over again, I need to remind my performance-based self that it's not about me. Just like in the story of Jairus's daughter, it was Jesus who was doing the healing. Indeed, He specifically told the girl, "Arise." He was the one! He did it. The little girl, lying there, didn't just all of a sudden, up and decide, *I'm getting up all by myself now.* How absurd, then, to think that I could do that as well? Once again, God showed me that He's patient—and that there's still more.

As God was making a lot of changes regarding my heart and my will, He still was working on my food, weight, and body issues. As grateful as I was to see the consistent 120 to 130 on the scale, in the end, I was learning it was just a number on a scale. It wasn't the sum total of who I was. God said, Himself, that He called me by name.

"Fear not, for I have redeemed you;
I have called you by your name;
You are Mine."
—*Isaiah 43:1*

I was more than this body, this face, a set of physical features. Being as focused and self-absorbed as I've been throughout my life, I'd become way too in touch with "me." Now, suddenly, from gradually, of all things, I'd wanted to want less of me in the picture—and more of Him.

"Jesus said to him, 'If you can believe,
all things are possible to him who believes.'"
—Jesus, in Mark 9:23

A **Prayer** to Rise

Father, I come to You in the name of Jesus, asking for help in my life. Thank You, Lord, that You can turn any situation around. There is nothing too hard for You **(Jeremiah 32:27).**

I ask You, Lord, to continually unfold my life before me. Change what is negative into positive results, fulfilling **Romans 8:28.** Help me to embrace Your Word being fulfilled.

Thank You for the miracles that have already taken place in my life, whether they be people or circumstances. And above all, thank You for the greatest miracle of all, Your Son, Jesus, my Savior. I gratefully accept Your love for me and I thank You with all of my heart. In Jesus's name, I pray. Amen.

Journaling Section

To Help You **Work Through** Your Thoughts

Who in your life do you consider to be part of your support system? Do you have a church family? Where do you feel a sense of belonging?

_____

_____

_____

_____

_____

_____

Think about **Romans 3:23**. How does that apply to your life and circumstances? How can you see yourself in a different light regarding this Scripture?

_____

_____

_____

_____

_____

_____

What are three healthy ways to deal with loneliness?

_____

_____

_____

_____

_____

_____

_____

_____

According to **Psalm 32:8,** God will instruct, teach, counsel, and watch over us. What things have happened in your life that demonstrate the reality of this Scripture?

_____

_____

_____

_____

_____

_____

_____

_____

Read **Psalm 37:4.** What are the desires of your heart? Have you asked God about them? If not, why not? What do you think would happen if you did?

_____

_____

_____

_____

_____

_____

_____

What are three kind things that someone has said to you? How did that make you feel?

_____

_____

_____

_____

_____

_____

_____

_____

List three specific traits you like about your physical appearance. Commit to complimenting or encouraging at least two people every day.

_____

_____

_____

_____

_____

Who are the positive, supportive people in your life?

_____

_____

_____

_____

Who are the negative, nonsupportive people in your life?

_____

_____

_____

_____

_____

How can you increase time spent with the positive influences and decrease time spent with the negative influences?

_____

_____

_____

_____

_____

_____

_____

_____

Consider **James 3:16**. What are the areas of "envy and self-seeking" in your life? How has it caused disorder? How can God help you change that?

_____

_____

_____

_____

_____

_____

_____

_____

Are your identity and sense of self and worth exclusively tied to your appearance? What else is valuable about you? Name three things and be specific.

_____

_____

_____

_____

_____

_____

_____

Hebrews 10:35–36 states that when we've done the will of God, we will receive what has been promised. First find in the Bible three Scriptures, three promises of something you want. Then ask God what His will for your life is concerning these Scriptures.

_____

_____

_____

_____

_____

_____

_____

_____

What discipline/correction has occurred in your life that was "for your own good"? How does **Proverbs 3:11–12** apply to your life now?

_____

_____

_____

_____

_____

_____

Do you feel solely responsible for fixing everything that's wrong? What do you think you can or should change?

_____

_____

_____

_____

_____

_____

_____

_____

_____

Using your own words, define the word *healed*. In your present situation in your life, what would healing mean to you?

_____

_____

_____

_____

_____

_____

_____

Do you believe that God can heal? Why or why not? (Refer to **Luke 5:12–13.**)

_____

_____

_____

_____

_____

_____

_____

_____

Read **Mark 9:23**. List everything in your life that you currently feel is "impossible." Then read that list to God in prayer. What would you like to have happen?

_____

_____

_____

_____

_____

_____

_____

Scriptures to Consider

Romans 3:23

Proverbs 18:24

Psalm 68:6

Isaiah 30:21

Psalm 32:8

Psalm 37:4

Proverbs 16:24

James 3:16

Luke 9:23–24

Psalm 139:14

1 Peter 5:7

Hebrews 10:35–36

Philippians 1:6

Proverbs 3:11–12

Proverbs 3:5–6

Job 5:17–18

Isaiah 53:5

Isaiah 42:1

Mark 9:23

Jeremiah 32:27

Philippians 4:8

What Is Recovery?

Recovery is much more than the abandonment of starving and stuffing. At minimum, it includes the following:

- Maintenance of normal or near-normal weight.
- In women, regular menstrual periods (not triggered by medication).
- A varied diet of normal foods (not just low-cal, nonfat, nonsugar items).
- Elimination or major reduction of irrational food fears.
- Age-appropriate relationships with family members.
- Awareness of cultural demands for unrealistic thinness.
- One or more mutually satisfying friendships with healthy, normal people. Such friendships involve mutual give-and-take and a minimum of caretaking and "parenting" behavior.
- Age-appropriate interest and participation in romantic relationships.
- Strong repertoire of problem-solving skills.
- Fun activities that have nothing to do with food, weight, or appearance.
- Understanding of the process of choices and consequences.
- Person has a sense of self, goals, and a realistic plan for achieving them and is moving toward building a meaningful, fulfilling, and satisfying life.
- Person has also learned to be kind to self and others, forsaking perfectionism and confronting flaws and disorder with grace and understanding. Person refuses to drive herself or himself with criticism and demands for unrealistic performance.

Adapted from ANRED, "Treatment and Recovery," http://www.anred .com/tx.html. Used with permission.

Taking Steps to Move Beyond Eating Disorders
(Author's Personal Advice)

- Accept God's love and forgiveness for you; He wants you to have this in your life.
- Forgive yourself and others. If struggling with forgiveness, ask God and others for help in coming to terms with it.
- Recognize the fact that the past is in the past, and that what happened there will not automatically mean that your future is not bright and hopeful.
- Engage in new opportunities, especially in meeting positive people.
- Find a church community with people and programs that can enrich your life.
- Explore your creativity: write in a journal, draw, paint, and dance. Expressing yourself through the arts is a wonderful, healing way to process issues in your life.
- Face your life head-on with honesty and courage. Even if you are scared.
- Be willing to learn about God and His Word, yourself, and the world around you. The learning process oftentimes sparks excitement, hope, purpose and a zest for life.
- Approach each day living in the moment, enjoying and making the most of the day God has given you.
- Approach life with faith and with a positive attitude. Whatever happens, God will always be there to help you through it.
- Practice the **Philippians 4:8** principle.

Chapter Ten

Ellipsis—
I'm Not There

I'm Not There

Somehow
in the middle of all of this,
Jesus
turned the impossible
into the achievable,
the doubts
into the believable,
Somehow
for now she's learned
No,
"I'm not there"
And that's her miracle from God,
Right there
Somehow
Jesus took her cliché glass
half empty and half full
and turned it into a cup for her,
"He restores my soul"
Yes,
God
is helping her to see that

"I'm not there"
It is the miraculous journey
not the impossible goal,
Water into wine,
Glass into cup,
God's love into whole soul,
"I'm not there"
It's no longer the discouraging of "so far to go" now,
It's inspiring
It's accomplishing now,
Somehow
in the middle of all of this
Jesus
turned the impossible defeat
into opportunity to meet
her
where she is right now,
It's all about perspective
and accepting
the incredible,
faithful
love
God wants to give
to this, to each little girl,
"He restores my soul"
"He restores my soul."

*"For I know the thoughts that I think toward you,
says the LORD, thoughts of peace and not of evil,
to give you a future and a hope."
—Jeremiah 29:11*

Two things I never thought I'd have: a future and a hope. "Yeah, that's great for you, Sheryle, but what about me?" Are you asking this question?

Let me encourage you, not by my words, but by God's Word. **"God shows no partiality"** (**Acts 10:34**). That means that His promises work just as much for you and apply just as much to you and your life as they do to me.

I want you to know, it's never too late. I don't care how far gone you think you are, how high or low you are on the scale. There is nothing that you've done or could ever do that will make God stop loving you.

*"For I am persuaded that neither death nor life,
nor angels nor principalities nor powers,
nor things present nor things to come,
nor height nor depth, nor any other created thing,
shall be able to separate us from the love of God
which is in Christ Jesus our Lord."
—Romans 8:38–39*

God loves you unconditionally. He doesn't love you any more or any less if you succeed or fail. He loves you because that is who He is by nature: "**God is love**" (**1 John 4:8**). And this love shows up in a number of different ways. One way is forgiveness.

"If we confess our sins,
He is faithful and just to forgive us our sins and
to cleanse us from all unrighteousness."
—1 John 1:9

"Therefore, if anyone is in Christ,
he is a new creation;
old things have passed away;
behold, all things have become new."
—2 Corinthians 5:17

God forgives, and because He loves you so much, He desires to forgive you of your sins. All you need to do is ask. That's all.

"For You, Lord, are good, and ready to forgive,
And abundant in mercy to all those who call upon You."
—Psalm 86:5

"Ask, and it will be given to you;
seek, and you will find;
knock, and it will be opened to you.
For everyone who asks receives,
and he who seeks finds,
and to him who knocks it will be opened."
—Jesus, in Matthew 7:7–8

God's unconditional love for you shows up in acceptance and approval. You are His beloved, beautiful, chosen daughter. He's already made up His mind about that. There's nothing you can do to change it.

"But God demonstrates His own love toward us,
in that while we were still sinners, Christ died for us."
—Romans 5:8

"You are My servant,
I have chosen you
and have not cast you away."
—Isaiah 41:9

You may not be feeling *any* of this right now. Trust me, the feeling part doesn't always come quickly and easily, but here's where I hope you can take comfort in another aspect of God's love: His patience.

*"Now may the God of patience and comfort
grant you to be like-minded toward one another,
according to Christ Jesus."
—Romans 15:5*

*"Love suffers long and is kind; . . .
bears all things, believes all things,
hopes all things, endures all things.
Love never fails."
—1 Corinthians 13:4, 7–8*

It's true—love never fails. And that is yet another part of God's love for each one of us. I want you to rest in this, because if you're going through any disordered eating patterns, it's probably a safe bet to say that you feel that you've failed yourself, God, your family—whomever. I want to let you know that we all blow it. That's part of being human. But God is beyond all of that. Don't worry; He knew exactly what He was getting into with you. He's not sorry He chose you. He is patient. He is unfailing.

*"Let us hold fast the confession
of our hope without wavering,
for He who promised is faithful."*
—Hebrews 10:23

*"Through the LORD's mercies we are not consumed,
Because His compassions fail not.
They are new every morning;
Great is Your faithfulness."*
—Lamentations 3:22–23

Of course, none of this means anything until it is personally experienced by you, the individual. And so, before I go any further, I'd like to invite you to personally experience this for yourself. And that can only come by accepting Jesus Christ as your Lord and Savior. This is where it all starts. This is where the answer, the healing for whatever you're going through starts: through a relationship with God as your Father, and with Jesus, God's Son, who loved, lived, and died for you, so you could experience this incredible relationship. Don't worry; you don't have to fix anything first. God will do the fixing. Just give Him your heart and mean it with *all* of your heart. If you haven't already accepted Jesus as your Savior, I invite you to do it now. Just pray the following prayer with me:

Jesus, I ask You to be the Lord and Savior of my life. I give my heart and life to you with all of my flaws and mistakes. I ask You to take me as I am, to forgive me, and to change me with Your Love. I accept that You died for me, and even though I may not understand all of the reasons why You did this for me, I thank You for it. Come into my heart, Lord Jesus, and take over my heart and life. Help me, heal me, and love me into being the daughter God has created me to be. Thank You for hearing my prayer and for saving me. Amen.

"The LORD your God in your midst,
The Mighty One, will save;
He will rejoice over you with gladness,
He will quiet you in His love,
He will rejoice over you with singing."
—Zephaniah 3:17

Congratulations! You are on your way! It's the best decision you'll ever make. And God will continue to help you make wise decisions. This leads me to another wonderful trait of God: His power.

"'Behold, I am the LORD, the God of all flesh.
Is there anything too hard for Me?'"
—Jeremiah 32:27

Yes, God's love for you is just the tip of the iceberg! Just think about that—your Daddy is an all-powerful God who can do anything! And He is the God of your flesh, whatever state that flesh is in. Let that sink in for a minute. God is relevant, personal, and capable of transforming anyone and anything! Having trouble? Still think you're beyond the point of no return?

*"The LORD your God, who goes before you,
He will fight for you."
—Deuteronomy 1:30*

*"But the Lord is faithful, who will establish you
and guard you from the evil one."
—2 Thessalonians 3:3*

*"'My grace is sufficient for you,
for My strength is made perfect in weakness.'"
—2 Corinthians 12:9*

Okay, so you have the Bible verses. You still may be thinking, "Now what? Where do I start?" I'm glad you asked.

Praying a prayer to receive Jesus is only the first step in the process, in this journey. You need to build from there.

You've already engaged in the first weapon in your arsenal when it comes to fighting this painful disorder: prayer. Sounds too simple? Believe me, prayer is powerful. Don't underestimate it. That's how you build your father/daughter relationship with God. Don't be intimidated by it. There is no one right way to pray. You'll get better at it as time goes by. Just be real with God. He knows everything anyway. Just talk to Him, it's that easy.

"Is anyone among you suffering? Let him pray."
—James 5:13

By developing your relationship with God through prayer, you will build a faith and trust in positive things. Meet God where you are, right here, right now. He will take care of your needs. He is a God of details. And He is your Father who loves you!

Praying is only one way to communicate with God. Studying God's Word, meditating, learning from other Christians, all become vital to your faith in God. You as a person, living in a corrupt world, have been exposed to and have been programmed into believing the lies of the devil. You need to connect with and learn all of the truth and wisdom that will empower you to become all that you can be. Advice from people, self-help books, and Internet sources can be wonderful aids in helping you become healthier, but you need to go to the source of all health and help: God's Word. Reading the Bible allows you to see God's heart, hear his voice. You are reading His words to you! And His words have transforming power for you personally, individually, uniquely.

Yes, God's Word definitely has power! And once you read and study it, you can recall it just when you need it—when you're in situations requiring wisdom and guidance. Suddenly, seemingly out of nowhere, you'll be reminded of a verse that applies to just your situation.

You can even pray Scripture verses! Once you know what God's heart is, what His Word says, you can pray those powerful promises for yourself! Not too shabby, huh?

> *"So shall My word be that goes forth from My mouth;*
> *It shall not return to Me void,*
> *But it shall accomplish what I please,*
> *And it shall prosper in the thing for which I sent it."*
> *—Isaiah 55:11*

Don't get intimidated by the size of the book or by the language. There are plenty of Bibles that are modern translations. And you can start small: Read a devotional that has one verse every single day. Read the Psalms. Read the Gospel of John. Just start reading, and sooner or later you'll find yourself enjoying it.

Another significant help is that of the Christian church community. You need to be in an atmosphere of love and support. Find a Christian church where you are taught about God: His love, His Word. Go to a church that teaches about Jesus: His life and death on the cross for our sins. Go to a church that is active, alive, and passionate about life and positive things.

Find a church that offers smaller groups for support. A lot of churches have large congregations, but one tool necessary for your health and happiness is connection with others on a one-to-one basis. If you can get plugged into a Bible study, great! This will nurture you spiritually, emotionally, and socially as you learn about God's love, Word, and people.

Seek out a trusted pastor or Christian counselor with whom you can share your thoughts and feelings. Eating disorders can carry a lot of baggage and unresolved issues that need to be addressed from God's loving perspective. This is a large part of the healing process. If you aren't ready yet to talk to a pastor or counselor, then confide in a family member or friend. Bottom line: The person should be trustworthy. This person should be on your side, be in agreement that God is a loving, healing God and Father, and have your best interest at heart. By pursuing a Christian perspective, you are better able to receive the love, grace, and forgiveness necessary to heal. Pray, seek God, and ask Him to reveal to you and send you the right person with whom you can openly share your heart.

An eating disorder is a powerful enemy. It seems to have a frightening grip on you and take control of your life. You may fear you will never beat it. But never forget who your Father is. He is more powerful than anything that comes against you.

> *"No weapon formed against you*
> *shall prosper."*
> *—Isaiah 54:17*

That's right, no weapon!

It's pretty overwhelming to look at one's life, to see all of the things that need changing and fixing. It can be overwhelming, especially when trying to get a handle on the issue of eating disorders. There seems to be a prevailing assumption that there is no cure; there's only coping.

"The LORD will perfect that which concerns me;
Your mercy, O LORD, endures forever;
Do not forsake the works of Your hands."
—Psalm 138:8

There may be some of you who are reading this who do not have eating disorders, but there is another addiction that is causing you pain and suffering. Addictions and compulsions can be to anything. It doesn't have to just be regarding things we can eat or drink. While it is true that alcohol, drugs, and food are often the first things that come to mind when we think of addictions, this is just a mere sampling. It is possible to become addicted to any substance, behavior, person, or thing. Addiction to anything takes the place that only God should occupy in our lives. Addiction is all about finding a God substitute, but addiction's *answer* is found in God.

At the end of the day, it does all comes back to God. You need to realize that there is an incredible God who will help you and guide you every step of the way in healing and changing.

That's the kind of hope I want to share with you. There is a life beyond eating disorders, when it's with God. It doesn't matter where you are on the scale, what you're struggling with, God is able. He's just waiting on you to be willing to accept Him to be able in your circumstances and life.

*"And we know that all things work together
for good to those who love God,
to those who are the called according to His purpose."*
—Romans 8:28

I never thought my life as it is now would have been possible. And I never would have dreamed that it was possible to have found, of all things, in my tangled mess of a life, my loving Heavenly Father. And I'm still finding Him, more and more. My life is the process of loving Him as His daughter. It is not perfect, but it is changing for the better, bit by bit. He's giving me more, more than what my little mind could ever conjure up.

*"Now to Him who is able to do exceedingly abundantly
above all that we ask or think,
according to the power that works in us,
to Him be glory in the church by Christ Jesus
throughout all ages, world without end. Amen."*
—Ephesians 3:20–21

Whereas once I had resigned myself to giving up and to death, I now have a passion for life. Whereas once, I was lying on the floor, collapsing not only in body but in spirit as well, I now, through Jesus, am rising. Jesus—the best gift a girl could ever receive from her Daddy.

Not everything in my life is tied up in a neat, perfect bow. I still have stuff to deal with concerning my family, my relationships, my attitudes, behaviors, etc. In fact, I'm currently dealing with the complexity of my father's death. He passed away in the summer of 2003. This has been a very difficult time for me to live through.

But I now know that I'm not alone. God is ever helping, ever guiding me through this incredible life He has given to me. My life has worth and value and is worth living. I don't need to be perfect in order to enjoy it. And neither do you! You just need a personal, loving father/daughter relationship with the greatest Father of them all.

Please, wherever you are, whatever hell you may be going through, know this: God is more loving, more powerful than your problem is, and He will get you past it. Just trust Him, turn to Him. Just trust Jesus to be your Savior and Lord. And just watch. You too, little girl, will arise!

"I will be a Father to you,
And you shall be My sons and daughters,
Says the LORD Almighty."
—2 Corinthians 6:18

"You received the Spirit of adoption
by whom we cry out, 'Abba, Father.'"
—Romans 8:15

I Went to Sleep (And Woke Up)

I went to sleep
Death
And woke up
Life,
I went to sleep
Old
And woke up
New,
Closed eyes and doors
Opened
and now
God
was in my sight,
I saw Him through Jesus,
I went to sleep
A broken
fat and thin
shell,
I woke up
A whole daughter,
It just goes to show you,
You never can tell
how God's love can raise you
from a deathbed,
Eyes and doors
closed
now opened
to Who
God is

and what
He's saying,
Eyes and doors closed
Now opened
to Him saying
Arise
Arise,
I went to sleep
Death
And woke up
Life,
I went to sleep
My own miserable hopeless own
And woke up
His beloved His,
I went to sleep
a dying girl
And woke up
God's daughter.

A **Prayer** to Rise

Father, I come to You in the name of Jesus, asking for help in my life. Thank You, Lord, for the hope that is in Your Word.

I ask You to work Your divine plan for my life. I recognize that Your Word is true and lasting, and that the promises in **Jeremiah 29:11** are for me—You plan to give me a future and a hope. Forgive me for doubting You and Your wonderful Word. I now choose to embrace You into my life.

Help me, Lord, to have patience for the continual work You are doing within me. I recognize that some miracles happen instantly and some take time. Help me to have the right attitude as I wait on You.

Thank You for being my loving Father and embracing me as Your daughter, no matter what. I thank You that You see me as Your daughter, not as a freak, a disorder, or a mistake. I renounce, in the name and by the blood of Jesus, all arguments, curses, disorders, and behaviors that are contrary to Your perfect plan for my life. I ask now that You, Lord, take their place in my healing process.

Thank You that even while I am this "work in progress," I am always Yours and You always love me as Your daughter. I receive this all now. I love You, Lord. In Jesus's name, I pray. Amen.

Journaling Section

To Help You **Work Through** Your Thoughts

Read **Jeremiah 29:11**. List below three things you want for your future.

_____

_____

_____

_____

_____

_____

_____

Using **Romans 8:38–39** as a guide, fill in the blanks as they relate to your life and situation.

For I am persuaded that neither _____,
nor _____, nor _____,
nor _____, nor _____,
nor _____, nor _____,
nor _____, nor _____,
nor _____ shall be able to separate us
from the love of God, which is in Christ Jesus our Lord.

What sins do you need to confess to God? Write them down and take them to God in prayer.

_____

_____

_____

_____

_____

_____

_____

Based upon **Romans 5:3–5** and **1 Corinthians 13:4, 7–8,** what are three areas in which you need patience concerning yourself and your situation?

_____

_____

_____

_____

_____

_____

_____

_____

According to **Lamentations 3:22–23**, God's mercies never fail and He is always faithful. List three ways God has been faithful/merciful to you in your life.

_____

_____

_____

_____

_____

_____

_____

_____

Read **2 Corinthians 12:9.** In what way(s) do you feel you are weak right now?

_____

_____

_____

_____

_____

_____

_____

Commit to and set aside a time of prayer with God. Write it down below and on a calendar.

_____

During that time, write whatever comes to your mind. Commit all of it prayerfully to God.

Read **John 5:39**. Commit to reading the Bible every day. Start with the book of **John** if you choose, but search the Scriptures, asking God to reveal His Word to you concerning your life right now.

_____

_____

_____

_____

_____

_____

_____

_____

_____

_____

_____

_____

_____

ThinEnough

Taking **Isaiah 54:17** into consideration, how has the situation/experience with food and weight been a "weapon" against you? How do you feel about what God says about that weapon concerning you?

_____

_____

_____

_____

_____

_____

Read **Psalm 138:8**. Write down any and all questions you'd like to ask God concerning your life's purpose. How can what you're going through now be used by God? Take these questions to God in prayer.

_____

_____

_____

_____

_____

_____

_____

Meditate on **Ephesians 3:20**, deliberately concentrating on positive blessings, goals, and dreams you want to see God do in your life. Write them down. Start out by meditating one to two minutes before you go to sleep, gradually lengthening the time.

_____

_____

_____

_____

_____

_____

Upon completing these exercises and questions, define what the word *arise* means to you and your life. Write this down as your "mission statement," and pray for God to help you experience this definition for yourself.

_____

_____

_____

_____

_____

_____

_____

Scriptures to Consider

Jeremiah 29:11	Acts 10:34–35
Romans 8:38–39	1 John 1:9
2 Corinthians 5:17	Psalm 86:5
Matthew 7:7–8	Romans 5:8
Isaiah 41:9	Romans 15:5
1 Corinthians 13:4, 7–8	Hebrews 10:23
Lamentations 3:22–23	Zephaniah 3:17
Jeremiah 32:37	Deuteronomy 1:30
2 Thessalonians 3:3	2 Corinthians 12:9
James 5:13	Isaiah 55:11
John 5:39	Isaiah 54:17
Psalm 138:8	Romans 8:28
Ephesians 3:20	Romans 8:15
2 Corinthians 6:18	Romans 5:3–5

New Hope® Publishers is a division of WMU®,
an international organization that challenges Christian
believers to understand and be radically involved in
God's mission. For more information about WMU,
go to www.wmu.com. More information
about New Hope books may be found at
www.newhopepublishers.com. New Hope books
may be purchased at your local bookstore.